Survive Sepsis
3rd Edition 2013 –2014

Author: Dr Ron Daniels
Publisher: United Kingdom Sepsis Trust.

FOREWORD BY DR RON DANIELS, CHIEF EXECUTIVE OF THE GLOBAL SEPSIS ALLIANCE:

Sepsis is one of our biggest killers: it claims 37,000 lives each year in the UK, leaving 65,000 survivors. Many of these survivors will have complications of sepsis, questioning 'why me?'. Direct costs to the NHS are around £2.5 billion per year. The good news is that you can help change this. The simplest interventions, including antibiotics and intravenous fluid challenges are more effective at saving lives than any currently available costly intensive care therapy. Rapid delivery of these interventions, which collectively we have termed the 'Sepsis Six', can also reduce long-term complications and save our healthcare system an estimated £160 million annually. All healthcare workers have a role to play in this, and this will become more important as sepsis becomes adopted as a clinical priority by NHS England in the next year. Survive Sepsis is an educational resource and tool kit compiled by juniors and edited by experts. Our team are here to ensure that you are equipped to recognise a patient with sepsis and act quickly to deliver the best care. Together, we can save an extra 12,500 lives a year in the UK.

Chief Executive of the Global Sepsis Alliance and UK Sepsis Trust

CONTENTS

INTRODUCTION

OVERVIEW

- Sepsis is the body's response to an infection. Systemic symptoms arise because the inflammatory response begins to affect the body's own tissues and organs.

- Sepsis is a huge problem, killing over 37,000 people a year in the U.K. and affecting a staggering 18 million across the globe annually.

- Sepsis is a continuum. Caught early, deterioration can be halted and if correct treatment is instigated the condition be reversed.

- Sepsis is everybody's problem! It can affect anyone, and can present to every medical specialty inside or outside hospitals, as well as developing whilst patients are in hospital for another reason.

- Sepsis care is best delivered as a team that includes nurses, doctors, physiotherapists or other health care workers. Being an effective member of this team makes a true difference to patients and their outcomes.

WHAT IS SEPSIS?

Is everybody with a temperature septic? Does everyone with a low blood pressure have septic shock?

Obviously the answer to these questions is 'no'; however, both of these subtle signs could signal the start of somebody developing sepsis. Keeping up your index of suspicion for sepsis could mean the difference between a patient's life or death. Our patients might be familiar with the older terms 'septicaemia' and 'blood poisoning', but an estimated 90% of our population have never heard of sepsis. Writing, and saying, 'sepsis' will gradually change this.

In some patients, sepsis can present with vague and non-specific symptoms, and only become really obvious when organs are beginning to fail. This, coupled with a historical lack of consensus on the definitions of sepsis, has affected our healthcare system's ability to spot sepsis and respond appropriately. We need to change this now.

THE DEFINITION OF SEPSIS:

Sepsis is a systemic response to a new infection. This means that the presence of a suspected or known infection with systemic manifestations (termed the 'systemic inflammatory response syndrome' or 'SIRS') defines sepsis.

Let's start with SIRS. When we cut our hand, burn our foot or bump our head, our bodies have the innate ability to respond to help us to overcome the injury. Inflammation starts- blood vessels dilate (termed 'vasodilatation'), and the capillaries 'leak' fluids. When this is localised, we see swelling around the injury due to water and other substances leaking out of the capillaries, and the area becomes warm and red due to the dilated blood vessels. This is protective- the increased blood flow means more white blood cells get to the area to fight any potential infection, and more platelets and fibrin are delivered to stop the bleeding. Capillary leakage is necessary because the damage is to the cells and tissues, and the white blood cells and other substances will do little good if they're stuck inside the blood vessels.

INFLAMMATION STARTS WITH VASODILATATION AND CAPILLARY LEAKAGE

Generalized inflammation manifests as SIRS. Our immune system is reacting fast- it signals for the bone marrow to make more white blood cells in case of infection and causes blood vessels to dilate. Our cells and tissues are working more quickly, and so the body needs more oxygen and glucose to help this increased workload (and to prepare us to run away from whatever caused the damage- an evolutionary response!). So patients with SIRS might have a high white blood cell count, a high temperature, a fast heart rate and respiratory rate, or a high blood glucose. The body can't keep this high level of response up forever- if whatever is causing the SIRS continues, some of these adaptive responses begin to fail. Our bone marrow might not be able to produce white blood cells as quickly as they're being used up if infection is present, and our white blood cell count might fall. Vasodilatation causes blood to be diverted to the skin and peripheries where we can lose heat, so our body temperature might begin to fall. This can also cause reduced blood flow to the major organs- our brain might not get enough glucose and oxygen, causing confusion, agitation or drowsiness.

This helps us to understand the definition of SIRS. The box below details the currently accepted criteria for SIRS- these were expanded from the 4 published by Roger Bone in 1992 after the first consensus definitions conference during a second consensus conference in 2001. If 2 or more SIRS criteria are present, then the patient has SIRS:

- **Temperature ≥ 38.3°C or ≤ 36°C**
- **HR ≥ 90 beats/min**
- **Respiratory Rate ≥ 20/min (or pCO_2 < 32mmHg)**
- **WBC count ≥12x10^9/l or ≤4 x10^9/l or >10% immature neutrophils**
- **Acutely altered mental state**
- **Capillary glucose > 7.7mmol/l in the absence of Diabetes Mellitus**

THE TEMPERATURE (AND THE WHITE CELL COUNT) CAN BE HIGH OR LOW IN SEPSIS

When the systemic inflammatory response is triggered by an infection (bacterial, fungal or possibly viral) then we class this as 'sepsis'. An infection doesn't need to be proven, just suspected. For example, if a patient has a productive cough with green phlegm, we suspect a chest infection. If another reports a burning sensation when passing water, we suspect a urinary tract infection. In a patient with a hot, swollen and tender joint, we suspect septic arthritis. Public awareness campaigns have taught us what to look for to suspect meningitis, but we know what other infections look like- if a patient is suspected to have an infection, we need to screen for sepsis,

As sepsis develops unchecked, the supply of oxygen and nutrients to the major organs can begin to fail, the inflammation can impair their function further by causing swelling and oedema, and/or their ability to compensate for the increased demand can begin to fail. Failure of any of the organs (lungs, kidneys, liver, heart and circulatory system, bone marrow, etc) denotes severe sepsis. Criteria for identifying severe sepsis will be dealt with in the next chapter.

BY THE TIME SEVERE SEPSIS HAS DEVELOPED, THE PATIENT HAS A 35% RISK OF DEATH

Septic shock is the most severe end of the sepsis spectrum. If an individual's blood pressure drops below <90mmHg systolic (or more than 40mmHg from their baseline) this is termed 'sepsis induced hypotension'. If we are then unable to remedy this blood pressure drop or organ failure with suitable intravenous fluid resuscitation, we class this as 'septic shock'.

It's important to remember that some patients can preserve their blood pressure even though the circulation is failing. This is still shock, but reliance on the blood pressure alone won't spot this group. Anaerobic respiration by the cells will cause lactic acid (lactate) to build up: a lactate of more than 4mmol/l at any time means septic shock is present. Severe sepsis and septic shock will be dealt with in more detail in the next section.

Septic shock carries a 50% mortality rate

DOES SEPSIS MATTER?

YES! Sepsis is a considerable burden on healthcare services throughout the world, with far-reaching human and economic costs. Not only does sepsis claim large numbers of lives (leaving many more bereaved and grieving), but it consumes over one third of Intensive Care resources and costs the NHS an estimated £2.3 billion per year in bed days. This is just the tip of the iceberg, though: for survivors, long term psychological and physical disability in as many as 1 in 5 patients can mean delayed return to work or early retirement, and ongoing demands on healthcare resources.

In the U.K. it is estimated that 37,000 people die a year as a result of sepsis. This number is alarming, yet even this number can hide the fact that sepsis mortality ranges from 35% in severe sepsis up to a staggering 50% in patients with septic shock. In comparison with other known 'killers' that are often seen in national advertising campaigns sepsis again stands out. In England and Wales during 2011 30,000 deaths were as a result of lung cancers, 24,500 as a result of COPD, 24,000 from heart attacks and around 20,000 from strokes. HIV caused 192 deaths over the same time period.

A patient with severe sepsis is one of the sickest patients you will ever see

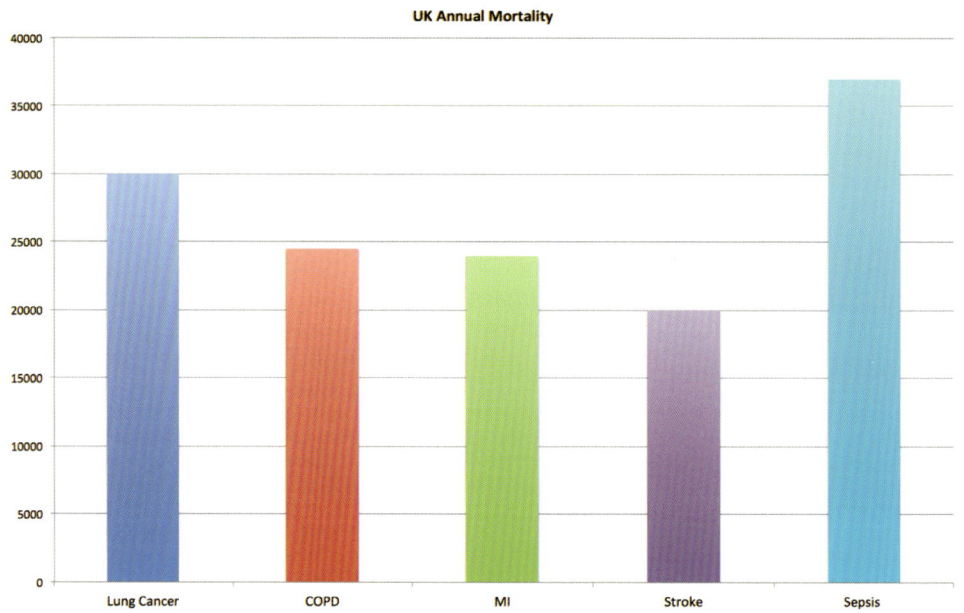

Scarily, sepsis is also becoming more common; in part as a result of years of antibiotic use and accompanying bacterial resistance, and in part due to our aging population with ever more complex co-morbidities. As a result, sepsis has sneaked into being one of the top 10 leading causes of death in the U.S. with an incidence that is rising by 1.5% a year. By 2020, we will be likely to see an extra 1 million cases a year!

Sepsis does not discriminate, affecting all ages groups in all health care settings including the community, prehospital and secondary care. Sepsis doesn't respect healthy lifestyle choices or social worth.   It can present on any health worker's watch, regularly crossing specialities and (though the majority of cases are community acquired) can rear its ugly head in those having a Healthcare-Associated Infection (HCAI).

Almost 30% of all patients admitted to an Intensive Care Unit (the most costly hospital beds) have sepsis or develop it within a day of being there. However, intensive care staff often do not see sepsis from its outset, and certainly won't be involved in all cases of sepsis. The huge array of presentations in a myriad of settings makes the 'ownership' of sepsis not one profession's or speciality's but one for all healthcare professionals. Having an index of suspicion, and recognising its subtle signs early, is of paramount importance provided treatment is then initiated immediately. As with other time critical conditions such as heart attacks or strokes, what we do in the first few hours of sepsis developing is critical to outcome.

Over the last 10 years, awareness of sepsis has risen, and screening tools to aid detection and 'care bundles' to guide early treatment supported by best evidence have been implemented in hospitals across the globe via the Surviving Sepsis Campaign. As a result, improvements have been made yet there is more work to be done. Compliance remains low and the process of care unreliable. In Emergency Departments in the UK in 2010, only 27% of patients with severe sepsis received antibiotics within an hour, and the figure for inpatients is likely to be significantly lower. We now need not only to fix hospitals' care delivery but also to move beyond a hospital focus and involve community-based and prehospital staff. The Global Sepsis Alliance, with partners including Survive Sepsis and the UK Sepsis Trust, are now addressing this need.

Observational studies have shown that patients receiving the basic aspects of care described by the Sepsis Six within 1 hour following recognition have a mortality reduction of nearly 40%: far in excess of the proposed 25% reduction aimed for by the Surviving Sepsis Campaign. The Sepsis Six empowers the non-specialist to contribute to the Surviving Sepsis Campaign's care bundles by delivering life-saving treatments earlier, and the truth is that these basic aspects of care, if delivered quickly, will save far more lives than any expensive, invasive intervention on intensive care.

RELIABLE, EARLY DELIVERY OF THE SEPSIS SIX WILL SAVE FAR MORE LIVES THAN EXPENSIVE TREATMENT ON INTENSIVE CARE

FIGURE 1 .THE RELATIONSHIP OF INFECTION, SIRS, SEVERE SEPSIS AND SEPSIS.

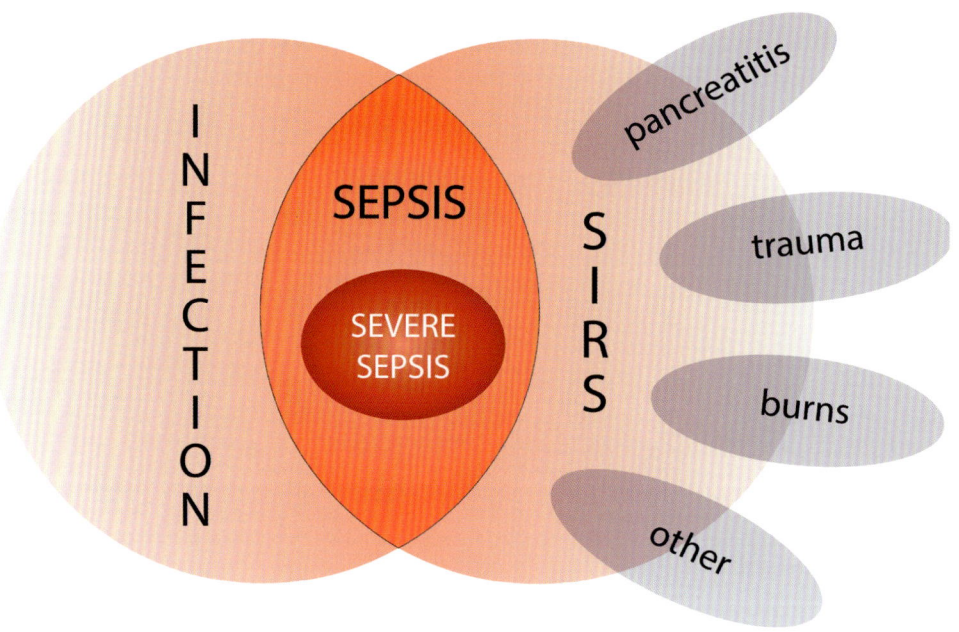

[ADAPTED FROM BONE RC ET AL. DEFINITIONS FOR SEPSIS AND ORGAN FAILURE AND GUIDELINES FOR THE USE OF INNOVATIVE THERAPIES IN SEPSIS. CHEST 1992; 101:1644-55]

SO WHAT CAN I DO?!

The SIRS response itself does not indicate the need for hospital admission, and some patients developing uncomplicated sepsis in the community can safely be kept at home with appropriate safety netting and review arrangements. Once severe sepsis has developed, though, hospital admission is mandatory and treatement becomes a medical emergency, so all patients suspected of having an infection or uncomplicated sepsis should be reviewed regularly.. Being the person who spots the signs of severe sepsis early and starts treatment withthe Sepsis Six, or gets help from someone who can, will truly make a difference, not only in lives saved but also by reducing the £2.3 billion cost of sepsis to the NHS annually.

The best way to deliver care is as a team whose members:

- Are aware of the condition
- Understand the need for early intervention and the consequences of delay
- Have open, clear lines of communication and can rely on each other to act as a team
- Can use a process, or care pathway that ensures elements of care are delivered at the right time
- Are committed to evaluating their performance regularly and continually looking for improvements

SEPSIS. SPOT IT. TREAT IT. BEAT IT.

FURTHER READING

Levy MM, Fink MP, Marshall JC, et al: 2001 SCCM/ ESICM/ ACCP/ ATS/ SIS International Sepsis Definitions Conference. Critical Care Medicine 2003; 31: 1250–1256

Sepsis- a guide for patients and relatives. The UK Sepsis Trust, 2013.

MacKenzie, I. Lever, A. Sepsis: definition, epidemiology, and diagnosis. British Medical Journal 2007; 335: 879

Martin G.S. et al. The Epidemiology of Sepsis in the United States from 1979 through 2000. New England Journal of Medicine 2003; 348:1546-1554

IDENTIFYING THE SEPTIC PATIENT

Which of these patients is septic?

A. A 78 year old man who has had flu-like symptoms for two days and has been taking regular paracetamol. His temperature is 37.0°C, his heart rate 100bpm and he hasn't passed urine in several hours.

B. A 18 year old woman with left flank pain and dysuria, a temperature of 38.7°C, a heart rate of 120bpm and a blood pressure of 82/43mmHg.

C. A 56 year old man who presents feeling generally unwell. He looks pale and is cold to touch with a temperature of 34. 0°C and a heart rate of 105bpm.

The answer is that all of them might be, and that each need evaluating for sepsis. With a high index of clinical suspicion and the use of a screening tool, septic patients are usually easy to identify. But sepsis continues to be missed, commonly with potentially devastating consequences. Early identification of septic patients and rapid initiation of the Sepsis Six saves lives.

This chapter will teach you which patients are most at risk of sepsis and why. You will learn to identify signs of sepsis, be introduced to a septic screening tool and learn how to apply it.

WHO IS AT RISK OF SEPSIS?

Any patient with an infection is at risk of developing sepsis, but certain groups are at a greater risk.

1. EXTREMES OF AGE

At both extremes of age people are more susceptible to infection and therefore to sepsis. Very young children have immature immune systems which may be unable to mount an adequate immune response to an infection. Elderly patients may have little physiological reserve to combat an infection. In each case the clinical signs and symptoms of sepsis may not be as pronounced, so a high index of clinical suspicion is vital.

## 2.	IMMUNOCOMPROMISED PATIENTS INCLUDING NEUTROPENIA

There are numerous causes of immunocompromise, some more severe in their effect than others (see table). Such patients cannot mount a sufficient response to an infection and localised infection can very quickly become systemic, leading to profound sepsis. Although their immune response (which triggers the inflammation causing organ dysfunction) is likely to be less aggressive than in non-immunocompromised patients, the problem is that the size of the infective insult increases rapidly- there are suddenly lots of bugs to trigger rapidly deteriorating sepsis. Such patients are also at risk of repeated and persistent infection; often with unusual organisms.

As with patients at the extreme of age, patients with a compromised immune system may not display such pronounced signs and symptoms of infection and high index of clinical suspicion is vital.

Strict aseptic technique is of the utmost importance when caring for immunocompromised patients. Patients should be reverse barrier nursed (and 'doctored'!!) to protect against organisms colonised on both healthcare staff and equipment. Universal precautions such as stringent hand cleaning, gloves, gowns and aprons should be used for every patient contact and equipment should be disposable where possible or patient-specific when not.

PRIMARY (CONGENITAL)

- INHERITED DEFICIENCIES E.G. B OR T CELL DEFICIENCIES
- INHERITED NEUTROPHIL DISORDERS: FAMILIAL NEUTROPENIA, CYCLIC NEUTROPENIA, AND INFANTILE AGRANULOCYTOSIS

SECONDARY (ACQUIRED)

- DRUGS: IMMUNOSUPPRESSIVE DRUGS SUCH AS CHEMOTHERAPEUTICS, DMARDS AND STEROIDS
- INFECTIVE CAUSES: SEPSIS, VIRAL ILLNESSES, HIV
- SEVERE ILLNESS INCLUDING TRAUMA AND BURNS
- POST RADIOTHERAPY
- MALIGNANCY
- SPLENECTOMY

SOME COMMON CAUSES OF IMMUNOCOMPROMISE

3. IATROGENIC PROCEDURES

Simple but vital invasive procedures like the insertion of central lines or peripheral venous catheters can leave patients at an increased risk of infection by breaking the natural defence barrier of the skin. Strict aseptic technique must be followed when inserting and handling indwelling devices including urinary catheters to avoid introducing infection.

Cannula insertion is an incredibly common procedure but simple steps such as skin cleaning according to local protocol, wearing gloves and using a sterile field substantially reduce risk of infection. It is important to regularly review a patient's need for a cannula and if it is not needed it should be removed immediately. All cannula insertion sites should be reviewed at least every 24 hours for signs of infection. Tools such a the Visual Infusion Phlebitis (VIP) score developed by Andrew Jackson are now widely used to support clinical decision-making in cannula management.

It would be rare for a patient to go through a hospital admission without at least one blood test, cannula or catheter. Each of these procedures has its own risk and careful consideration should be given as to whether the procedure is in the patient's best interests.

Surgical procedures such as laparotomy cause more obvious disruption to the body's natural defence systems. With this in mind, a large number of patients will be started on prophylactic broad-spectrum antibiotics when undergoing major surgery. The decision to prescribe these must be based on a risk/ benefit analysis for the particular procedure and patient. There is a current trend toward reducing the number of procedures for which prophylactic antibiotics are routinely used, and local protocols are usually available to guide prophylaxis.

Although the above have been highlighted as risk factors for the development of sepsis it is important to remember that nearly all patients fall into at least one at risk group. By the very nature of being unwell and the hospital environment itself, inpatients are at an increased risk. So-called "superbugs" such as MRSA and C.difficile have caused many deaths over recent decades, although the incidence of such infections is falling, and antibiotic resistance is becoming a major concern with some organisms now sensitive to only one class of antibiotic.

IDENTIFYING THE SEPTIC PATIENT

The approach to assessing any unwell patient is always the same – following the ABCDE approach. Identifying and treating immediately life-threatening conditions as you thoroughly and sequentially assess the patient is of primary importance. Care specific to the septic patient should follow this immediate assessment and will complement it.

THE SCREENING TOOL:

This is an example of a screening tool used for identifying sepsis in hospital. Many such examples exist, and will vary according to clinical area and population (for example, those used by Paramedics will not include investigations available only from a laboratory). Using the sepsis screening tool in any acutely unwell patient can quickly alert you to the fact that your patient is septic and that you need to act quickly as this is a medical emergency. This screening tool has two parts – firstly you assess the patient for the SIRS criteria and secondly to assess for the signs of infection.

THE SEPSIS SCREENING TOOL SHOULD BE APPLIED WHEN A PATIENT:

- is admitted, or transferred to a new clinical area, with a diagnosis consistent with an infection.

- triggers on a track-and-trigger warning system, such as NEWS or MEWS (National Early Warning Score, Modified Early Warning Score)

- deteriorates during treatment for another condition or after an intervention

- fails to improve as expected, for example post-operatively

- whenever you are worried about a patient- trust your 'sixth sense'!

Between one third and one half of episodes of inpatient deterioration are caused by a pre-existing or new infection...

Apply if MEWS is 4 or more, or if infection suspected

Are any **2** of the following SIRS* criteria present and new to your patient?

Obs:	Temperature <36 or > 38.3°C ☐	Respiratory rate > 20/ min ☐
	Heart Rate > 90 bpm ☐	Acutely altered mental state ☐
Bloods:	WCC < 4 x10⁹/l or > 12 x10⁹/l ☐	Glucose > 7.7 mmol/l ☐ (if patient is not diabetic)

If patient is *neutropenic* and any 1 present, follow 'yes' and call Consultant

Follow standard MEWS protocol
Re-apply screening tool if situation changes

NO 🟥 **YES** 🟩 Tick appropriate box

Patient has SIRS: Think SEPSIS!!!! Call FY or CT doctor using SBAR Situation: 'Suspected Sepsis'

Is this likely to be due to an infection?
For example

Cough/ sputum/ chest pain ☐	Dysuria ☐
Abdo pain/ distension/ diarrhoea ☐	Headache with neck stiffness ☐
Line infection ☐	Cellulitis/ wound infection/ septic arthritis ☐
Endocarditis ☐	

NO 🟥 Tick appropriate box **YES** 🟩

Patient has **SIRS***

Continue MEWS every 30 mins
Give oxygen to keep SpO₂>92%
Consider fluid challenge
Look for other causes of SIRS
(pancreatitis, transfusion reaction, trauma, burns, thromboembolism)
Re-evaluate for sepsis if MEWS increases or condition changes
Discontinue screen

This patient has SEPSIS
Ensure Doctor present within 30 mins
Immediately start Sepsis Six Pathway
(overleaf)

| Time of SBAR call: | Doctor's name: | Referring staff name: |
| | | |

(* SIRS = Systemic Inflammatory Response Syndrome)

1. THE SIRS CRITERIA

SIRS stands for systemic inflammatory response syndrome and is characterised by 2 or more of the following physiological and laboratory parameters*:-

- **Temperature ≥ 38.3°C or ≤ 36°C**
- **HR ≥ 90 beats/min**
- **Respiratory Rate ≥ 20/min (or pCO_2 < 32mmHg)**
- **WBC count ≥12x10⁹/l or ≤4 x10⁹/l or >10% immature neutrophils**
- **Acutely altered mental state**
- **Capillary glucose > 7.7mmol/l in the absence of Diabetes Mellitus**

One of the causes of SIRS is sepsis and that is why the screening tool starts with an initial assessment of the patient looking for the SIRS criteria.

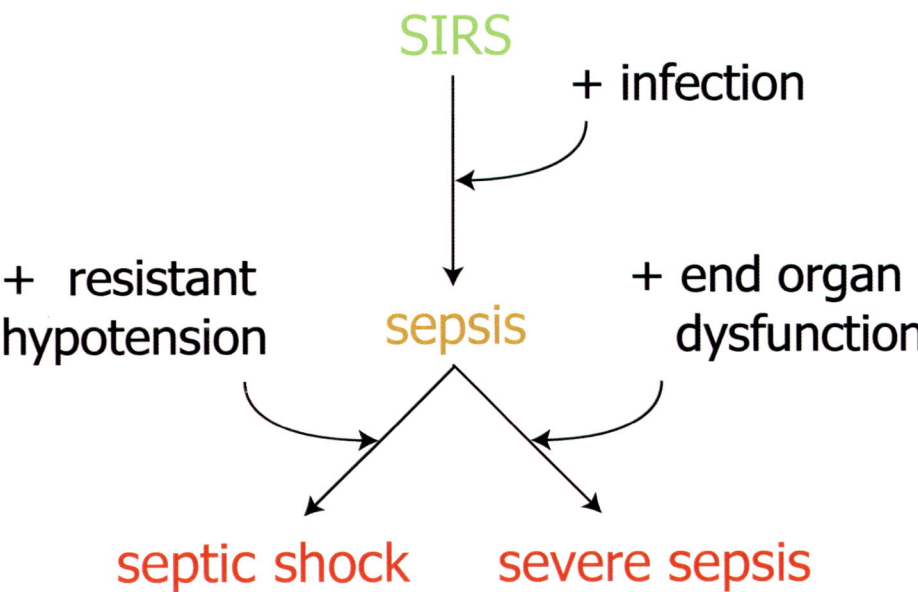

*ORIGINALLY, 4 SIRS CRITERIA WERE DESCRIBED AT A CONSENSUS DEFINITIONS CONFERENCE IN 1991 (PUBLISHED 1992). THIS CONFERENCE WAS REPEATED IN 2001, AND RESULTED IN AN EXTENSIVE LIST OF AROUND 30 CRITERIA. THE 6 CRITERIA USED NOW WERE ADAPTED BY THE SURVIVING SEPSIS CAMPAIGN FROM THIS EXTENDED LIST.

Temperature (<36.0°C or >38.3°C):

A high temperature (in our screening tool) is one that is above 38.3°C and a low temperature is one that is below 36.0°C .

It is important to remember that septic patients can be both hyper- and hypothermic. Some patients, who have taken anti-pyretic agents such as paracetamol and ibuprofen, may have a normal temperature when you assess them.

Pyrogens (substances which cause altered body temperature), both produced by the body (endogenous) and released by microbes (exogenous), lead to the release of a molecule called prostaglandin E2. This has an effect on the hypothalamus, the temperature control centre of the body. The result is a disruption in the body's normal thermoregulatory systems, and leads to a rise in overall body temperature.

As sepsis develops, blood vessels increase in diameter and therefore volume. This vasodilatation leads to an increased peripheral blood volume and a correspondingly warm and pink appearance. Vasodilatation also contributes to hypotension and compensatory tachycardia, but can also lead to increased heat loss from the peripheries: this can eventually lead to a drop in core body temperature.

In the later phases of sepsis, the peripheral circulation will shut down and the skin become cool and mottled. Hyperacidaemia due to poor perfusion only compounds this, and other factors reduce the heart's ability to pump blood effectively, so patients can become cold and pale with poor capillary refill.

Tachycardia (> 90bpm):

Both the pyrogens released in sepsis and the body's immune reaction to it lead to an increase in metabolic activity, resulting in an increase in oxygen demand throughout the tissues.

Oxygen is delivered to cells throughout the body via the bloodstream, carried by haemoglobin molecules in red blood cells (though as described in the Sepsis Six chapter, small amounts are dissolved in plasma). As the oxygen demand of cells increases, the body attempts to meet this demand by raising cardiac output. One of two ways of increasing the cardiac output is to increase the heart rate, explaining why patients who are septic are often tachycardic. The other means of increasing cardiac output is to increase stroke volume, as demonstrated by the equation below.

If the supply of oxygenated blood cannot keep up with demand the patient becomes shocked.

Definition of shock - Tissue perfusion which is not adequate for the body's metabolic requirements

CARDIAC OUTPUT = HEART RATE X STROKE VOLUME

CARDIAC OUTPUT = THE AMOUNT OF OXYGENATED BLOOD IN ML LEAVING THE HEART PER MINUTE

HEART RATE = THE NUMBER OF TIMES THE HEART BEATS PER MINUTE

STROKE VOLUME = THE VOLUME OF BLOOD EJECTED FROM THE VENTRICLE WITH EACH CONTRACTION

As mentioned previously, in profound sepsis vasodilatation is a frequent occurrence. When the small arteries and veins dilate, the volume of blood they can carry substantially increases. However, there is no extra fluid to fill this space so the amount of blood returning to the heart will decrease- this is known as 'relative hypovolaemia' (See Sepsis Six chapter). This results in the amount of blood ejected by the heart with each beat, the stroke volume, being reduced. However the body still needs to increase the cardiac output to meet the metabolic demands, so demands a large increase in heart rate occurs to compensate for these changes. This tachycardia is only a temporary fix though; the compensation can only last so long before the heart muscle begins to tire.

Increased Respiratory Rate (>20):

Tachypnoea is best defined as an abnormally high respiratory rate for an individual patient. The definition of a 'normal' respiratory rate varies, but a respiratory rate of more than 20 is seldom normal in adults. Respiratory rate is one of the most sensitive signs of an acutely unwell patient and therefore one of the most important to measure correctly. If you measure this over 15 seconds, an error of one is made four times greater when scaled up. Measuring over one full minute can be time well spent.

As discussed above, in sepsis the oxygen demand of tissues throughout the body increases. This increased demand can be met in one or both of the following ways:

1. **By increasing the amount of oxygenated blood being delivered to the end organs (by increasing cardiac output, giving rise to a tachycardia)**
2. **By increasing the amount of oxygen in each ml of blood being delivered to the tissues**

In order to adequately oxygenate the increased amount of blood circulating through the lungs due to attempts by the body to increase cardiac output, the respiratory rate increases.

Patients with severe sepsis may have tachypnoea for reasons other than to increase oxygen availability and delivery to the tissues. Pneumonia may be the source of sepsis; patients can develop pulmonary oedema as a result of the inflammatory process, or an acute lung injury or the Acute Respiratory Distress Syndrome can develop. Each of these may occur alone or in combination. Each will cause a degree of hypoxaemia (reduced oxygen tension in the arterial blood) which in turn stimulates an increased respiratory rate. These conditions can also increase the work of breathing- it becomes harder for the respiratory muscles to bring about inspiration and expiration. This ultimately causes further tachypnoea as the patient fatigues, because the volume of air taken in with each breath reduces (low tidal volumes) and respiratory rate increases in an attempt to prevent a rising carbon dioxide. The overall effect is for the breathing to become rapid and shallow.

Hypotension:
Hypotension in sepsis is defined as a systolic blood pressure of less than 90mmHg, a mean blood pressure of less than 65mmHg, or a drop of more than 40mmHg from the patient's usual systolic blood pressure.

The change in blood pressure associated with sepsis is intrinsically related to the other physiological changes which occur, and is due to a combination of vasodilatation, fluid loss from capillary walls and an as yet undefined compound which directly reduces cardiac output.

The mean arterial pressure is the average pressure throughout the cardiac cycle, and gives us a good indication of pressure available for end organ perfusion.

Mean arterial pressure = Diastolic pressure + (Systolic-Diastolic)/3

Sepsis causes a drop in the systemic vascular resistance by causing vasodilatation, leading to a proportionate decrease in effective circulating volume (more intravascular space without an increase in fluid to fill it) - a 'relative' loss of intravascular volume or 'relative hypovolaemia'.

As sepsis develops, the inflammatory overreaction and cascade leads to changes in the way capillaries work. They become so compromised that instead of retaining fluid they 'leak' into the surrounding tissue. This leakage contributes to the massive oedema which is commonly seen in severely septic patients. This leakage of fluids can also lead to a further reduction in the effective circulating volume leading to a further fall in blood pressure- an 'absolute' loss of intravascular volume or 'absolute hypovolaemia'.

When a patient is hypotensive as a result of sepsis and don't respond quickly to IV fluids they are in shock. It is vital that this is recognised quickly and treated aggressively – as highlighted in the Sepsis Six chapter.

Acutely altered mental state

Patients who are septic may be confused or agitated and may even be delirious. GCS of less than 15 or an acute decrease in GCS may alert you to the fact that this patient may be septic. The acute alteration in mental state is due to a combination of factors including disruption of the blood brain barrier and disturbance of cerebral autoregulation (the way in which blood flow to the brain is regulated) due to the systemic inflammatory response. Shock and hypoxia will also lead to an altered mental state. This may be a symptom that family members or carers report and it is vital to include sepsis in the differential diagnosis of any patient who has an acutely altered mental state. Patients are commonly described as 'looking drunk', 'slurring their speech' or just 'not being right'. It is vitally important to listen to such 'soft signs'.

WBC count ≥12x10^9/l or ≤4x10^9/l or >10% immature neutrophils

Although both a high and a low white cell count are included as one of the SIRS criteria, initially the white cell count may not be known. You must not delay treatment whilst awaiting blood results; instead you should treat based on clinical suspicion. Patients with sepsis can have both a raised or a low leucocyte (white cell) count. The majority of patients develop a leuocytosis (high white cell count) as a natural host response to the infection. Patients may also have an increased percentage of immature neutrophils due to enhanced bone marrow activity, so-called 'left shift'.

However, some septic patients may also have a low white cell count. This is vital to remember as patients who are immunocompromised may not be able to mount a good immune response to infection and can deteriorate quickly. In some cases, a low white cell count is a late sign: early in their sepsis state they may have had a high count, but as the sepsis progresses the bone marrow may not be able to keep pace; it can't produce enough white cells to replace those being consumed. This is an ominous, late sign. Of particular concern are patients who are known to be or at risk of being neutropenic. These patients, who may be on immunosuppressive therapy such as chemotherapy, need to be identified early and treated aggressively according to neutropenic sepsis guidelines.

Hyperglycaemia in the absence of Diabetes Mellitus (Capillary glucose >7.7 mmol/L)

Hyperglycaemia may be found initially in the septic patient as part of the 'stress response' and is due to multiple factors. The stress response releases substances into the bloodstream aimed at mobilizing glucose: it's also know as the 'flight or fight' response and is an evolutionary mechanism to allow us to run away from injury. These factors include an initially low level of circulating insulin, high level of cortisol and high levels of glucagon, all of which contribute to hyperglycaemia. A capillary blood glucose of over 7.7 mmol/L in the absence of a diagnosis of diabetes mellitus forms one of the SIRS criteria and all acutely unwell patients need a capillary blood glucose check as part of their initial assessment.

2. SIGNS AND SYMPTOMS OF INFECTION

Once an assessment for the SIRS criteria has been made the next step is to assess the patient for signs and symptoms of an infection. This requires a brief but comprehensive screen for any potential source of infection combining history taking and an examination of the patient.

Is this likely to be due to an infection?

For example

Cough/ sputum/ chest pain	☐	Dysuria	☐
Abdo pain/ distension/ diarrhoea	☐	Headache with neck stiffness	☐
Line infection	☐	Cellulitis/ wound infection/ septic arthritis	☐
Endocarditis	☐		

Sepsis is a time critical medical emergency and it may be difficult at the time to pick up on the source of infection immediately but the most vital thing is to treat sepsis aggressively by using the Sepsis Six and try to identify the source of infection. However, identification of the source of infection must not delay antibiotic therapy.

History taking is vital - the patient's history may not only help you to identify the source of infection but it very quickly alert you to the fact that they might be septic. Patients may report that they feel extremely unwell and the worst they ever have felt when poorly. It is therefore vital to listen to your patient when taking their history and pick up on these clues to the diagnosis. This will be covered further in the common presentations chapter.

SEPSIS. SPOT IT. TREAT IT. BEAT IT.

FURTHER READING

Daniels R, Nutbeam T (Eds). The ABC of Sepsis.
Chichester, Wiley-Blackwell books, 2010

THE SEPSIS SIX

OVERVIEW

1. Delivering the Sepsis Six within one hour is one of the most effective life-saving treatments in medicine

2. Each hour's delay in giving antibiotics increases mortality by 7.6% (in septic shock)

3. The Sepsis Six aims to measure and corrects problems with oxygen delivery

4. Always assess the impact of your treatment and adjust accordingly

---

THE SEPSIS SIX

Step 4:
Give fluids

Step 3:
Give antibiotics

Step 2:
Take cultures

Step 1:
Give oxygen

Step 5:
Take Hb & lactate

Step 6:
Monitor urine
output / catheterise

INTERVENTION	WHY?
Give oxygen	*To prevent a low haemoglobin saturation from worsening O_2 delivery*
Take blood cultures	*To help select appropriate antibiotics when results back*
Give antibiotic	*To treat the underlying problem*
Give fluid	*To prevent a low circulating volume from contributing to hypotension and reducing cardiac output*
Take Hb/lactate	*Hb > to ensure a low Hb is not worsening O_2 delivery* *Lactate > to check for inadequate oxygen delivery, which suggests severe sepsis*
Take hourly urine output	*To monitor fluid balance*

INTRODUCTION

In the previous chapter, we saw how sepsis can ultimately cause multi-organ failure and death. In this chapter, we will see how applying the Sepsis Six works to minimise this.

The Sepsis Six is a set of six (!) tasks which can be performed by any junior health professionals working together as a team. It is simple and effective, and has been shown to greatly increase a patient's chances of survival if delivered within the first hour.

The Sepsis Six should be delivered as quickly as possible, but always within the first hour following recognition of sepsis.

STEP ONE: GIVE HIGH FLOW OXYGEN

Your septic patient is in a state of high oxygen demand. This means we need to maximise oxygen delivery.

There are a few equations coming up to explain why we do what we do. Rest assured you do not need to memorise them for clinical practice.

Oxygen delivery is governed by two things: how much oxygen is in the blood, and how much blood is flowing to the tissue or organ. Writing this as an equation gives:

O_2 delivery = O_2 content of blood x cardiac output

The O_2 content of blood is then given by this equation:
Oxygen content/ml = [1.34 x [Hb] x % sat] + 0.003 x pO_2

Let's break down this equation to see how it relates to the Sepsis Six.

[Hb] is the concentration of haemoglobin in g/dL (note some hospitals use g/L). We will go further into this in Step 5: Take [Hb] and Lactate.

The **% sat** (oxygen saturation of haemoglobin) is the amount of oxygen bound to haemoglobin as a percentage of the total amount of oxygen that could potentially be bound to haemoglobin.

Each gram of haemoglobin can carry up to 1.34ml of oxygen. If each gram of haemoglobin were instead carrying 1.25ml of oxygen, the oxygen saturation would be:

$$\frac{1.25}{1.34} = 93\%$$

In other words, **% sat measures how full of oxygen the haemoglobin is**.

Blood has multiple gases in it. Each gas makes a contribution to the total pressure. The partial pressure of oxygen (pO_2) refers to the contribution of oxygen to the total pressure.

In our equation opposite, **pO_2 (partial pressure of oxygen in the blood)** refers to the pressure exerted by oxygen in the blood.

HOW IS OXYGEN CARRIED IN THE BLOOD?

Oxygen is transported in two forms:

1. **the amount of oxygen bound to haemoglobin – this is really important (98% of total oxygen carried)**

2. **the amount of oxygen dissolved directly in the blood - this is relatively unimportant (2% of total oxygen carried)**

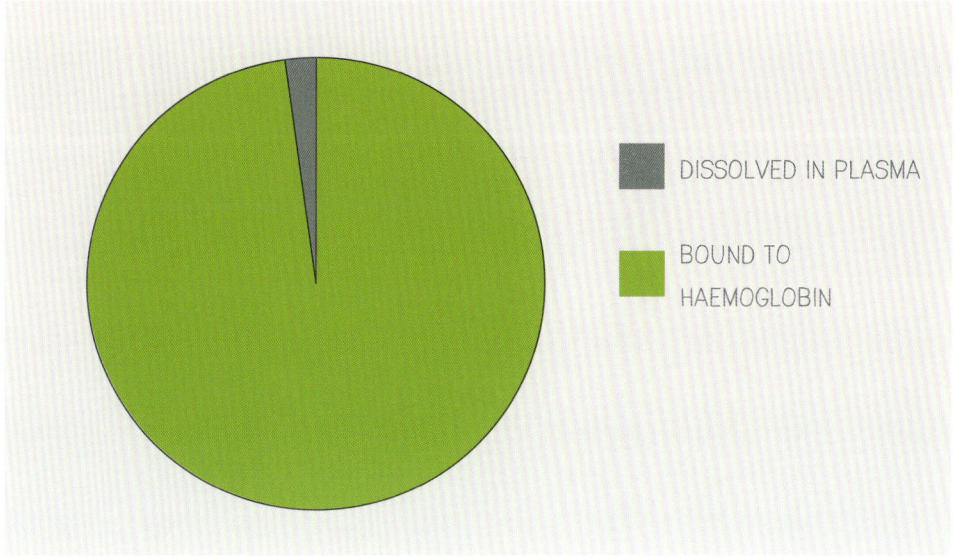

DISSOLVED IN PLASMA

BOUND TO HAEMOGLOBIN

This is reflected in the earlier equation:

$$\text{OXYGEN CONTENT/ML} = [1.34 \times [\text{HB}] \times \% \text{ SAT}] + 0.003 \times PO_2$$

$[1.34 \times [\text{Hb}] \times \% \text{ sat}]$ is the amount of oxygen bound to haemoglobin.

$0.003 \times \mathbf{pO_2}$ is the amount of oxygen dissolved directly in the blood.

This means that what we really want to focus on is maximising the [**Hb**] x **% sat**. Since we can't change the constant 1.34, and since the amount of oxygen dissolved in plasma is minimal, for practical purposes the oxygen content equation can be simplified as:

Oxygen content $\approx$ [**Hb**] x & **% sat**

The only practical way to maximise oxygen content is to ensure that there's enough haemoglobin to carry oxygen, and the haemoglobin is well saturated with oxygen.

[Hb] will be dealt with in Step 5: Take [Hb] and lactate.

The effect of a high or low pO_2 beyond its effect on % sat is very limited. This means that % sat gives you all the information you are likely to need about whether or not pO_2 is adequate for your patient.

In other words, you only need to specifically check pO_2 on an arterial blood gas if you cannot get a reliable % sat trace with the pulse oximeter: e.g. peripherally shut down, certain arrhythmias, carbon monoxide poisoning etc. For most situations, the pulse oximeter is more than adequate for assessing oxygenation.

Of course, you will need blood gas results for other reasons e.g. quick lactate, pH, pCO_2 etc. In most situations, a venous blood gas is as useful as an arterial stab.

There are some factors beyond pO_2 which play a role in determining % sat, which you can read about below the graph if you are interested.

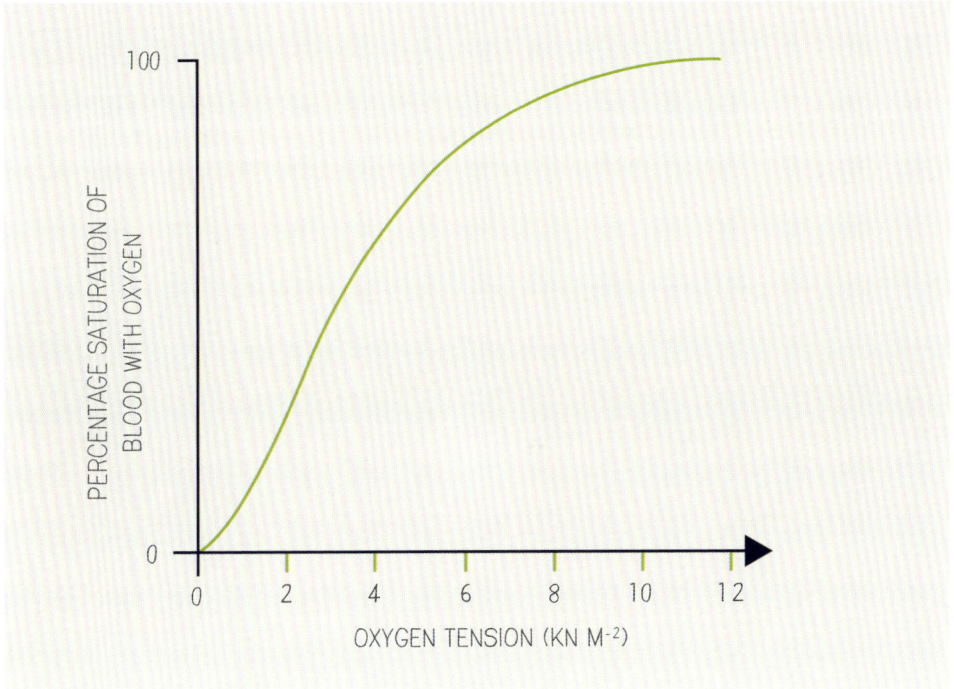

Those other factors...

The exact shape of this curve will vary with other factors like temperature, pH, and pCO_2. High temperature, low pH and high pCO_2 are all potential markers of high metabolic activity/oxygen demands, and produce a shift in the curve to the right. This shift encourages haemoglobin to unbind from oxygen more readily, which releases more oxygen into the tissue. This helps deliver oxygen to the tissues where it is most needed. Physiologically, the main effect of these variables is to assist oxygen unloading, with more oxygen released to the most metabolically active tissues.

KEY POINT

THE % SAT LARGELY DETERMINES THE OXYGEN
CONTENT OF THE BLOOD FOR A GIVEN [Hb].

HOW INCREASING THE AMOUNT OF INSPIRED OXYGEN CAN INCREASE THE OXYGEN DELIVERED TO THE TISSUES

---

1. Increasing the fraction of oxygen (FiO_2) in the inspired air with a face mask increases the amount of oxygen in the alveoli

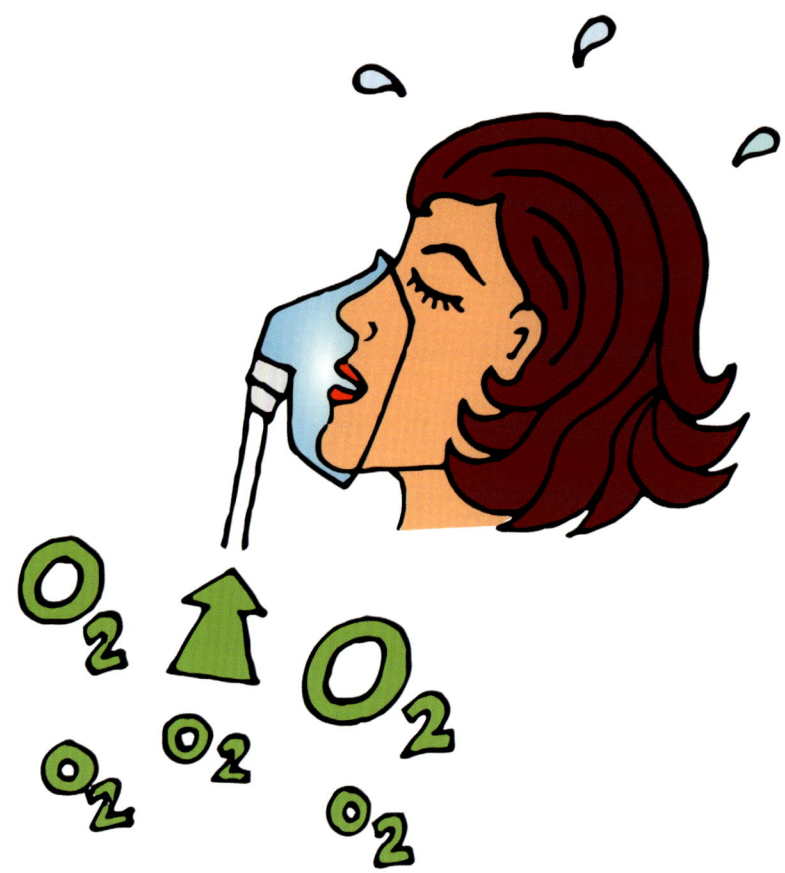

2. The extra oxygen in the alveoli encourages more oxygen to diffuse across into the blood in the lungs

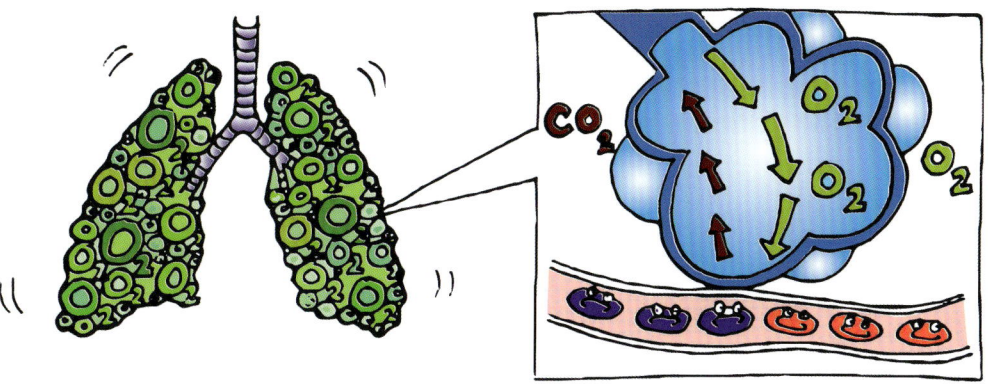

3. The extra oxygen is mostly carried by haemoglobin in red blood cells, which increases the oxygen content of the blood reaching the tissues

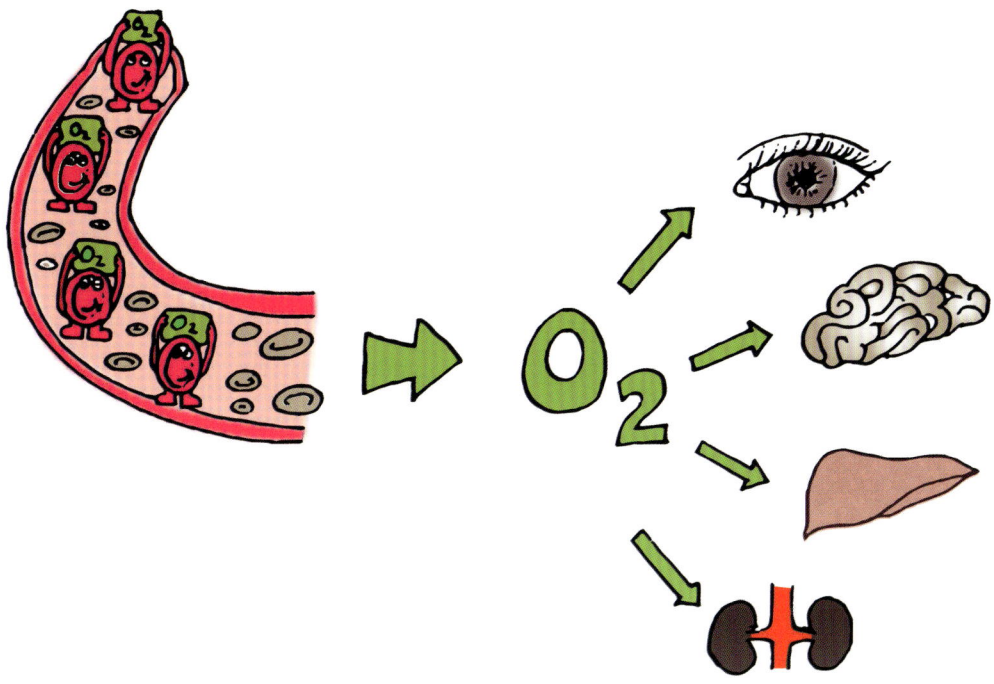

WHAT ARE THE BENEFITS OF OXYGEN?

Increasing the amount of inspired oxygen in a patient with low saturations, for example, <94% (check with your local policy on oxygen administration) will increase the oxygen content of the blood, which will increase the delivery of oxygen to tissues.

This is important as there is a critical imbalance between oxygen supply and demand in sepsis. In practice, during the early resuscitative phase the administration of high flow oxygen is usually appropriate in all patients. This includes patients with COPD. The British Thoracic Society (BTS) guidelines for the delivery of oxygen acknowledge this need in the patient with sepsis. Once the resuscitative phase is over (which usually corresponds to completion of the Sepsis Six with no evidence of septic shock, improving indices such as lactate and urine output and no other organ dysfunction) oxygen should be titrated to achieve saturations of 94-98% in most patients. In patients with known COPD, seek senior advice and have a low threshold for repeating arterial blood gas sampling. Once the oxygen saturations are at 98%, there is little benefit in further increases in the amount of inspired oxygen.

KEY POINT

Increasing the inspired oxygen will increase oxygen saturations, which increases the oxygen content of the blood.

Above a saturation of 98% there is little benefit from further increases in oxygenation.

WHAT ARE THE RISKS OF OXYGEN?

There is a small risk of hypercapnic respiratory failure.

Normally blood in the lungs flows to the alveoli (air-filled sacs where gas exchange occurs) that are best ventilated. The way the body works this out is by the amount of oxygen in the alveoli. A low amount of oxygen in an alveolus leads to less blood perfusing that alveolus by narrowing the capillaries supplying it with blood- this is known as 'hypoxic pulmonary vasoconstriction'. This means that the best performing parts of the lung receive most of the blood. Thus, CO_2 is easily removed, as most of the blood will go to alveoli that are ventilating well and so will be effective at removing CO_2.

When high flow oxygen is given, all the alveoli become better oxygenated, and so blood is spread more evenly through the lung rather than focused on the best performing, well ventilated areas. This means that CO_2 removal becomes less efficient. For most people, this is not a problem, as we can increase our tidal volume and respiratory rate to remove this extra CO_2. This theory has largely replaced the theory of hypoxic drive in explaining hypercapnia developing in patients with COPD who are given high flow oxygen.

In patients with limited ventilation ability, this can result in them retaining CO_2. These patients are at risk of hypercapnic respiratory failure, and include:

1. **Some COPD patients (particularly those on home oxygen or with previous hypercapnic respiratory failure)**
2. **Patients with neuromuscular problems affecting their breathing**
3. **Patients with chest wall/spinal deformities**
4. **Very obese patients**
5. **Patients with bronchiectasis, including secondary to cystic fibrosis**

Hypercapnic respiratory failure is dangerous as it can lead to respiratory acidosis. It must be remembered that hypercapnia leading to acidosis generally happens slowly, and that regular blood gas monitoring can identify this. Hypercapnia can be managed with controlled oxygen, NIV and/or invasive ventilation. Multi-organ failure from hypoxia happens quickly and rapidly becomes a problem that requires HDU/ITU or even becomes irreversible. In other words, hypoxia will kill quicker than hypercapnia.

For patients at risk of hypercapnic failure, close liaison with a senior doctor is essential (Specialist Trainee level and above in the UK) and/or senior nurse with specialist skills (e.g, a Respiratory Nurse Specialist). The aim will generally be to give the highest tolerated amount of inspired oxygen.

One pragmatic approach, though not grounded in an evidence base, is to target oxygen saturations of 94-98% in these groups. You can then re-check a blood gas (if the pulse oximeter is working well, venous is acceptable) at 30 minutes. If their CO_2 remains normal continue, whereas if it has risen consider the need for ventilation or reduce target range to 88-92%.

KEY POINTS

1. THERE ARE A SMALL GROUP OF PATIENTS AT RISK OF HYPERCAPNIC RESPIRATORY FAILURE WITH HIGH FLOW INSPIRED OXYGEN.
2. EVEN IN THESE PATIENTS, HYPOXIA WILL KILL BEFORE HYPERCAPNIA.
3. IN GENERAL, THE HIGHEST TOLERATED OXYGEN FLOW SHOULD BE SOUGHT, WITH BLOOD GASES TO CHECK FOR CO_2 RETENTION AND ACIDOSIS.
4. SENIOR MEDICAL AND NURSING INPUT SHOULD BE SOUGHT FOR THESE PATIENTS.

PRACTICAL TIP: SO HOW SHOULD WE OXYGENATE THE PATIENT?

Specific guidance is available in the BTS Guidelines for sepsis:

1. THE INITIAL OXYGEN THERAPY IS A RESERVOIR MASK AT 15 L/MIN.

2. ONCE THE PATIENT IS STABLE, REDUCE THE OXYGEN DOSE AND AIM FOR TARGET SATURATION RANGE OF 94-98%

3. IF OXIMETRY IS UNAVAILABLE, CONTINUE TO USE A RESERVOIR MASK UNTIL DEFINITIVE TREATMENT IS AVAILABLE.

4. PATIENTS WITH COPD AND OTHER RISK FACTORS FOR HYPERCAPNIA WHO DEVELOP CRITICAL ILLNESS SHOULD HAVE THE SAME INITIAL TARGET SATURATIONS AS OTHER CRITICALLY ILL PATIENTS PENDING THE RESULTS OF BLOOD GAS MEASUREMENTS, AFTER WHICH THESE PATIENTS MAY NEED CONTROLLED OXYGEN THERAPY OR SUPPORTED VENTILATION IF THERE IS SEVERE HYPOXAEMIA AND/OR HYPERCAPNIA WITH RESPIRATORY ACIDOSIS.

Patients should not receive dry, high flow oxygen for more than 4-6 hours due to the risks of retained secretions, dehydration and loss of heat. If a patient continues to require high inspired oxygen concentrations then this must be humidified.

STEP TWO: TAKE CULTURES

Cultures are essential to identify the organism causing sepsis and its sensitivities, and hence rationalise therapy.

Blood cultures should be taken percutaneously, and from all intravenous access devices that have been in for more than 24 hours (i.e, take more than one set if an intravenous device is in place).

Cultures should be taken before antibiotics are started, unless this would significantly delay the time to the first antibiotic dose. The only exception to this rule is in patients with purpura fulminans- the characteristic rash seen in meningococcal and streptococcal disease. If you see this, give antibiotics without delay!

There is a direct relationship between the blood volume in the culture bottles and the yield, with an approximately 3% increase in yield for every ml of blood. In the UK, 8-10ml of blood should be in each blood culture bottle. If you are struggling to get sufficient blood from the patient, do not unduly delay antibiotic therapy to obtain cultures.

PRACTICAL TIP:
IF YOU CAN ONLY GET A LIMITED AMOUNT OF BLOOD, ADEQUATELY FILL THE AEROBIC BOTTLE BEFORE FILLING THE ANAEROBIC BOTTLE, AS THE VAST MAJORITY OF ORGANISMS CAUSING SEPSIS WILL GROW IN THE AEROBIC BOTTLE.

IT'S NOT JUST ABOUT BLOOD CULTURES...

If you suspect a source of sepsis, send other body fluids too: for example sputum, urine, CSF, or any overt pus. The more samples the lab receives, the greater the chance of identifying the bug. This can help your patient in one of two ways: if the bug is resistant to the antibiotics you have chosen, you can change to the right therapy more quickly, and if it is a sensitive organism you can change to a less toxic, narrower spectrum agent and reduce the risk of causing a secondary infection.

STEP THREE: GIVE ANTIBIOTICS

KEY POINT:

EACH HOUR'S DELAY IN GIVING ANTIBIOTICS IN SEPTIC SHOCK
IS ASSOCIATED WITH A 7.6% INCREASE IN MORTALITY.

Antibiotic choice should be guided by the suspected focus of infection. This depends on your clinical, microbiological and radiological evidence for infection.

The choice of antibiotic should be in line with your local hospital guidelines; if in doubt, discuss with the microbiology and infection control teams.

SEPSIS, NOT SEVERE AND WITHOUT SEPTIC SHOCK

If you are confident about the source of the infection, then the antibiotic choice should be tailored to cover the likely pathogens according to local antibiotic prescribing guidelines.

If you are less confident about the source of the infection, then a broad spectrum covering gram negatives and gram positives can be started. It may well be appropriate to commence oral antibiotics in uncomplicated sepsis, but it is always sensible to speak with a senior first.

The choice and need for antibiotics should be reviewed daily and also as soon as culture and sensitivity results are known in order to reduce antibiotic resistance and toxicity.

SEVERE SEPSIS OR SEPTIC SHOCK

Patients with severe sepsis or septic shock should receive broad-spectrum therapy intravenously. This should be de-escalated as soon as culture and sensitivity results (check after 48 hours) are known in order to reduce resistance and toxicity.

PRACTICAL TIP: TRUST YOUR LOCAL EXPERTS

YOUR TRUST WILL HAVE A LOCAL ANTIBIOTIC POLICY, DEPENDING ON THE SOURCE OF THE INFECTION. THE COMMONEST TWO SOURCES ARE CHEST AND ABDOMINAL INFECTIONS, SO A BROAD SPECTRUM β LACTAM, WITH OR WITHOUT AN AMINOGLYCOSIDE AND WITH CONSIDERATION TO ANAEROBIC COVER, ARE GOOD STARTING POINTS.

Responsible antibiotic stewardship involves reviewing the decision to keep the patient on IV antibiotics at 24 and 48 hours. Discussion with microbiology can be very helpful here.

STEP FOUR: GIVE FLUIDS

Fluids are key to ensuring that the tissues get the oxygen and nutrients they need: helping to restore the imbalance between oxygen supply and demand.

To start with, consider again how oxygen delivery to the tissues is determined:

$$O_2 \text{ DELIVERY} = O_2 \text{ CONTENT OF BLOOD} \times \text{CARDIAC OUTPUT}$$

... or, the amount of oxygen delivered to a tissue or organ depends on how much oxygen is in the blood, and how much blood is flowing to the tissue or organ.

CARDIAC OUTPUT

The cardiac output is one of the determinants of oxygen delivery to tissues and organs. There are two factors governing cardiac output:

CARDIAC OUTPUT = STROKE VOLUME X HEART RATE

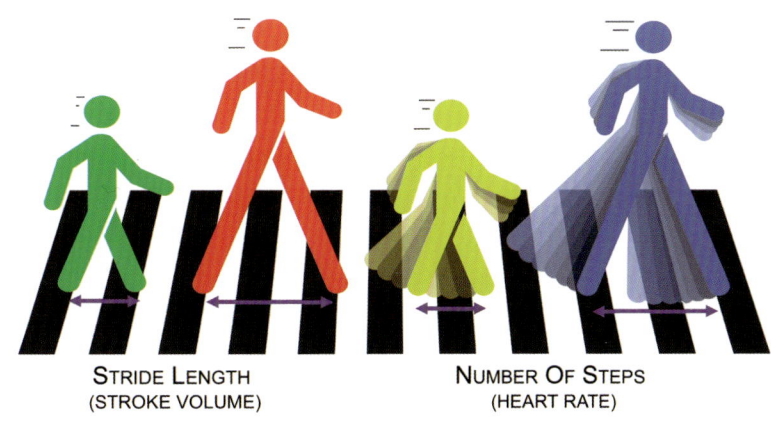

STRIDE LENGTH
(STROKE VOLUME)

NUMBER OF STEPS
(HEART RATE)

COMBINED = CARDIAC OUTPUT

Diagram above: Your walking pace is given by the length of your stride multiplied by the number of strides per minute. In a similar way, cardiac output is given by the stroke volume multiplied by the heart rate.

The body will naturally increase the heart rate in an attempt to overcome a low blood pressure or vasodilatation- this effect is frequently seen early in sepsis.

The stroke volume is dependent on three variables:

1. Preload

'Preload' describes how 'full' the heart is before it contracts to eject blood- it's determined by the circulating volume. A hypovolaemic patient will have a low preload and a low stroke volume.

Greater circulating volume → Increased venous return → Increased force of contraction → Increased stroke volume

The reason the increased venous return leads to increased force of contraction is because of the Frank Starling mechanism. This states that the more blood that stretches the heart whilst it is filling, the more forcefully it contracts. (See figure opposite)

In a healthy heart, preload is often the major determinant of stroke volume.

2. Afterload

This is the pressure that the ventricle must overcome to eject blood, caused by the tone (state of contraction) of the blood vessels, and is otherwise known as the 'systemic vascular resistance'.

A higher afterload leads to a reduced stroke volume because the heart has to work harder to overcome the resistance. In sepsis, the afterload is usually low, and the heart rate and contractility (see below) will need to increase to maintain cardiac output.

In non-septic patients with heart failure, afterload is often a major determinant of stroke volume. In sepsis, the afterload is often low, and so contractility becomes the main determinant of stroke volume in sepsis with heart failure.

3. Contractility (inotropy)

This is how hard the heart is contracting. It is increased by sympathetic stimulation, which is the body's natural response to a low blood pressure. In patients with heart failure, there is a limit to how hard the heart is able to contract. This means that patients with heart failure do not compensate well for vasodilatation.

In septic patients, the effective circulating volume is often decreased. This is due to a combination of relative hypovolaemia (same amount of circulating volume but occupying a bigger space) and absolute hypovolaemia (reduced circulating volume):

Relative hypovolaemia is caused by blood vessels dilating (vasodilatation). Even if the circulating volume stays the same, the bigger space it has to fill means the circulation behaves as though it has lost volume. Vasodilatation is the biggest cause of circulatory failure in previously healthy patients with sepsis. Its effect can be partly reversed by giving intravenous fluids to correct the relative hypovolaemia.

Adequate filling

Myosin filament (does not move)

Actin filament (does move)

Cardiac muscle contracts by the 'walking' of actin filaments over myosin filaments in response to calcium release. When the heart muscle is adequately stretched by 'filling', there is plenty of room for molecular movement and contraction is strong.

Underfilled

When the heart is empty, the actin and myosin have little room to move over each other. Contraction is weak and stroke volume, and therefore cardiac output is limited.

Overfilled

Here the heart is overfilled to the extent that there is no overlap between actin and myosin - the filaments can't 'grip' each other. Contraction is extremely weak and cardiac failure results.

Absolute hypovolaemia occurs for two reasons::

A. a lack of total body fluid, or

B. body fluid in the wrong place.

LACK OF TOTAL BODY FLUID

This can be from decreased intake of fluid, or increased fluid losses. Some causes are given in the table:

FLUID	INCREASED LOSSES
Lack of appetite	Sweating
Lethargy	Increased ventilation
Confusion	Diarrhoea
Decreased consciousness	Vomiting
	Bleeding (DIC)

FLUID IN THE WRONG PLACE

When fluid is in the wrong place, this usually means fluid has moved from the plasma into the tissues, so it's no longer in the circulation

For fluid to remain in the blood vessels requires two things:

1. **The forces encouraging fluid to stay in the vessels must be greater than the forces encouraging fluid to leave the vessels**

2. **The blood vessels must not be leaky**

The first point is based on Starling's law of the capillaries. This states that the hydrostatic and oncotic pressure differences between the blood vessels and tissue compartment are the driving force of fluid movement between these compartments.

Hydrostatic pressure is what we're used to measuring- if the blood pressure is 120/60 in a leaky blood vessel, and the pressure in the tissues around it is 20mmHg, fluid will tend to leak out of the vessel into the tissues. Oncotic pressure, on the other hand, is a pressure caused by the amount of proteins in the space. Fluid tends to stay in the space containing proteins, particularly albumin. Thus, if the patient has a low level of albumin, more fluid will tend to leak out of the vessels into the tissues.

The second determinant- leaky blood vessels- is particularly relevant in sepsis. In sepsis, the infectious organism triggers the release of multiple inflammatory messengers or 'cytokines'. The target for these inflammatory messengers includes the inner lining of the blood vessels (endothelium, particularly in capillaries), where they cause them to leak. As described in a previous chapter, capillary leak is a healthy response when localized to a site of injury, but harmful when it is generalized. Capillary leak will increase whenever there is alteration, damage, or death of the endothelial cell.

KEY POINTS

The aims of fluid therapy are:

1. to correct absolute and relative hypovolaemia

2. to bring the patient's pulse, blood pressure and urine output within target

3. to do this judiciously, and to avoid pushing the patient into overload

THE SEPSIS SIX

FLUID CHOICE

Crystalloids are the preferred first line fluid for resuscitation.

An appropriate initial fluid in most patients is Hartmann's solution.

FLUID	ADVANTAGES	DISADVANTAGES
Hartmann's	1. 30% of fluid remains in intravascular space 2. Not associated with hyperchloraemic metabolic acidosis	1. Contains potassium, so make sure the patient is not potassium overloaded 2. Caution in liver disease- Hartmann's contains small amounts of lactate which can accumulate
0.9% Sodium chloride	1. 30% of fluid remains in intravascular space 2. Does not contain potassium, so may be safer in established renal failure without urine output	1. Risk of hyperchloraemic acidosis if high volumes given
5% dextrose	1. None (in the acutely hypovolemic patient)	1. Only 10% of fluid remains in the intravascular space: poor at replenishing circulating volume 2. Can cause hyponatremia
Colloids (except allbumin)	1. As for 0.9% sodium chloride	1. Starch solutions carry a risk of acute kidney injury compared to crystalloids
Albumin	1. Stays predominantly in the vasculature. Consider when large volumes of resuscitation fluid needed. SAFE study suggestive of benefit in sepsis	1. Very expensive
Packed red cells	1. Corrects anaemia and stays in vasculature	1. Risks of blood transfusion 2. Crossmatched blood not immediately available 3. Contains a lot more potassium than Hartmann's!

In the early stages of sepsis ('warm sepsis'), a previously healthy patient typically 'looks' well perfused- vasodilatation mean that their peripheries are pink and warm, and their cardiac output is preserved or higher than normal as they increase their heart rate and contractility. Don't be fooled, though, their blood pressure might be already lower than ideal, and these patients will still need guided fluid resuscitation to correct their relative hypovolaemia.

Later in sepsis, the relative hypovolaemia becomes compounded by absolute hypovolaemia. Patients begin to become puffy with oedema as capillaries begin to leak fluid into the tissues, and ultimately their compensatory mechanisms will not be able to keep pace with the losses. Their body attempts to compensate by shutting down peripheral perfusion- the skin at the peripheries becomes cool and clammy, and sometimes takes on a 'mottled' appearance. This is sometimes known as 'cold sepsis', and means the patient needs urgent and aggressive resuscitation. The situation can be made even worse by circulating factors reducing contractility of the heart in sepsis.

RATIONALISING HOW THE FLUIDS ARE GIVEN

Imagine a tank full of fluid attached to a pump. After the pump there's a valve to boost the pressure of the fluid coming out (like when you put your thumb over the end of a hosepipe to boost pressure). There's a thirsty Ms Pacman which is relying on this fluid to keep herself hydrated.

If Ms Pacman is dried out, this is analogous to inadequate perfusion of the tissues, which is shock.

If a patient is in shock, this means this could be because of a lack of fluid (hypovolemic shock). In our Ms Pacman situation, the pump can't work properly as it can't draw enough fluid. Cardiogenic shock means a lack of pumping power: in Ms Pacman's plight, the pump is failing and the flow of water is low. In distributive shock, which includes septic shock, vasodilation means that although blood flow might be high, pressure is low and the cells distant from the capillaries won't receive any oxygen. Here, Ms Pacman is standing just too far away from a wide-bore hose: the flow is good, but the low pressure means the water falls to the floor at her feet.

The things we measure can give us clues as to where the problem lies. The 'markers of end organ perfusion' tell us if the patient is in shock.

Their conscious level may become affected as their brain perfusion reduces. A fall in perfusion to the kidneys can cause a low urine output. Perfusion to the peripheries can reduce later in sepsis (described above) and will result in a delayed capillary refill. Poor global perfusion can be assessed by measuring blood lactate, since anaerobic metabolism causes the production of lactic acid.

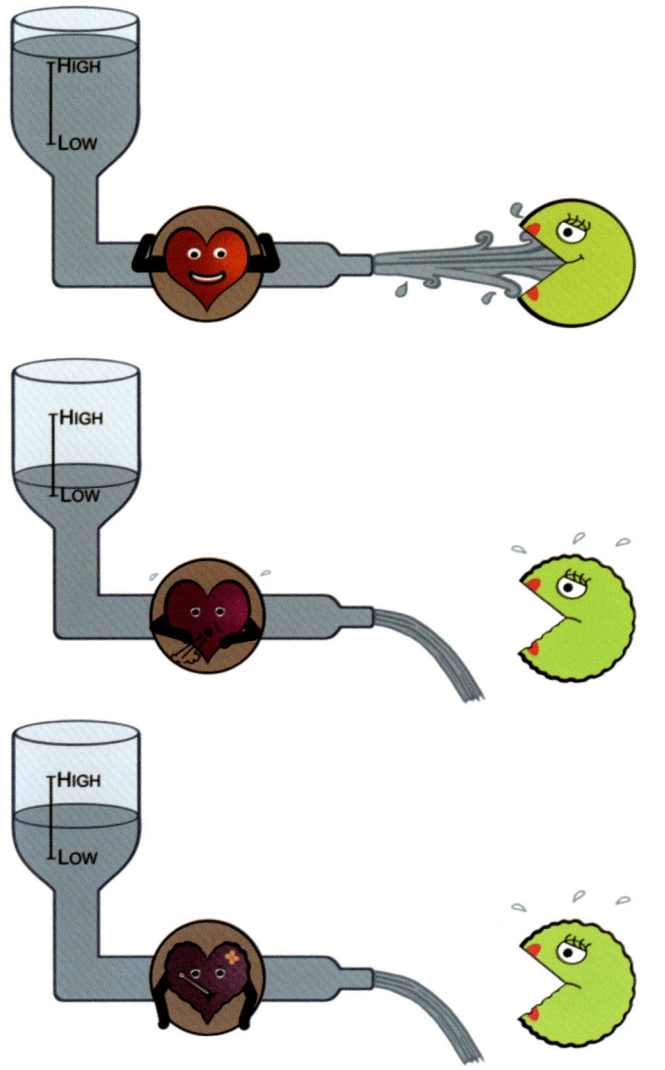

NORMAL BLOOD VOLUME, NORMAL CARDIAC FUNCTION AND NORMAL PERIPHERAL PRESSURE MEANS GOOD END ORGAN PERFUSION

A HYPOVOLEMIC STATE LEADS TO POOR END ORGAN PERFUSION, EVEN IF THE CARDIAC FUNCTION IS NORMAL.

POOR CARDIAC FUNCTION LEADS TO POOR END ORGAN PERFUSION, DESPITE AN ADEQUATE BLOOD VOLUME

Blood pressure is an important measurement, but a low blood pressure doesn't actually prove the patient is in shock, in much the same way that a low pressure at the valve is not proof that Ms Pacman is dehydrated. To find this out, we have to look at Ms Pacman directly and assess the markers of end organ perfusion.

This also means that a high blood pressure is not proof that a patient is not in shock, in much the same way that a high pressure at the valve does not prove that Ms Pacman is well hydrated.

The bottom line is that each patient is different, and some patients will be in shock at blood pressures that others would tolerate with no problem. Whilst a very low blood pressure is likely to cause inadequate perfusion in all patients, we must be careful not to be reassured by a BP of 109/61 when the capillary refill is 4 seconds, for example.

TO MEASURE CAPILLARY REFILL (BASED ON THE ALS GUIDANCE)

APPLY CUTANEOUS PRESSURE FOR FIVE SECONDS ON A FINGERTIP HELD AT HEART LEVEL (OR JUST ABOVE) AND COUNT THE TIME IT TAKES FOR CAPILLARY REFILL AFTER THE PRESSURE HAS BEEN RELEASED. THE NORMAL VALUE FOR CRT IS USUALLY LESS THAN TWO SECONDS.

Ideally, we would be able to see the blood pressure, pulse, urine output, lactate production and capillary perfusion change in real time as we give the fluid to help judge the amount and rate required.

In practice, we cannot measure these parameters continuously on the ward. However, we can measure the pulse, blood pressure and urine output at specific times, and capillary refill is a useful bedside clinical sign.

This is where the idea of a fluid challenge comes from. On the ward, the goal is to improve the haemodynamic markers that we can measure by giving repeated fluid challenges until there is no further improvement or until there are signs of fluid overload.

In sepsis, early aggressive fluid resuscitation improves the outcome. The initial total volume in patients with evidence of poor perfusion should be at least 30ml/kg, delivered as quickly as possible and certainly within the first hour. This can be delivered in divided fluid challenges of 500ml of crystalloid or 300 ml of colloid, provided that there is a favourable response after each challenge.

A typical fluid challenge would be prescribed as:

FLUID	DRUGS ADDED	DOSE	VOLUME	RATE
Hartmann's	-		*500ml*	*STAT*

(FOR A 60 KG PATIENT WITH NO RISK FACTORS FOR FLUID OVERLOAD; REMEMBER WE WOULD BE AIMING TO GIVE UP TO 1800ML IN THE INITIAL RESUSCITATION PERIOD FOR THIS PATIENT)

Scenario

Ms Margerie Jowelbottom is a 65 year old woman who has had a fever for the past day and has experienced burning on passing urine for the past two days. She is SIRS positive and a urine dipstick is positive for nitrites and leucocytes.

Her obs on admission are:
Pulse 102
BP 99/78
RR 22
Sats 100% on air
Temp 38.5
(Weight = 70 kg)

Clinically, she has a capillary refill of 3 seconds and her lips seem dry. Her chest is clear, and there is no peripheral oedema.

The catheter has drained 30ml of dark urine.
You are awaiting the blood results.

Your team has already performed five of the Sepsis Six, and has asked you to manage the fluids.

In this scenario, you should prescribe a fluid challenge.

FLUID	DRUGS ADDED	DOSE	VOLUME	RATE
Hartmann's	-		*500ml*	*STAT*

Remember we would be aiming to give up to 2100ml in the initial resuscitation period for this patient depending on response

20 minutes later, her observations are:
Pulse 90
BP 113/82
RR 20
Sats 100% on air
Temp 38.6

The catheter has drained a further 20 ml in this time.

There are three key questions to ask yourself after each fluid challenge:

1. **Is the patient showing any signs of fluid overload?**
   If overloaded, stop giving fluids and consider the need to offload fluids e.g. loop diuretic.

2. **Have the pulse, blood pressure and urine output responded favourably?** If they have not responded favourably, look for causes for these markers other than hypovolemia. It is also possible that they are severely hypovolemic.

If they have responded favourably, proceed to question 3

3. **Where is the MAP, pulse and urine output in relation to my targets?** If they have responded and the markers are acceptable in relation to your targets, then stop fluid resuscitation for now, although you must regularly reassess the patient

If they have responded favourably but the markers are still not acceptable in relation to your targets, repeat the fluid challenge.

The targets for the blood pressure, urine output and temperature are:

1. **Mean Arterial Blood Pressure > 65mmHg**

The mean arterial pressure is the diastolic pressure plus one third of the 'pulse pressure' (difference between systolic and diastolic). This is because the heart tends to spend approximately twice as much time in diastole (relaxation) as in systole (contraction)

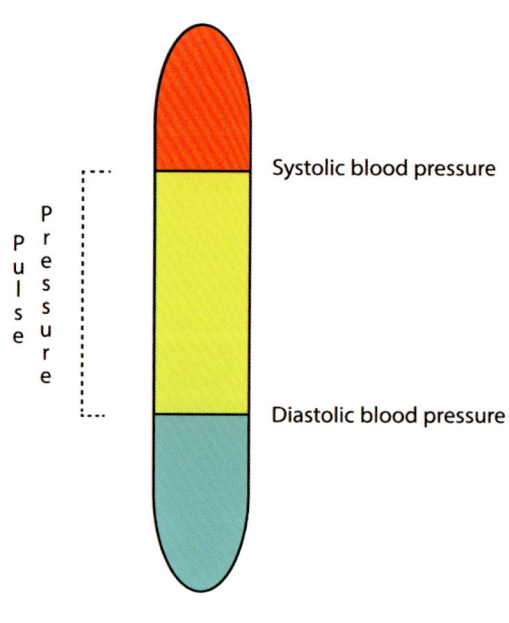

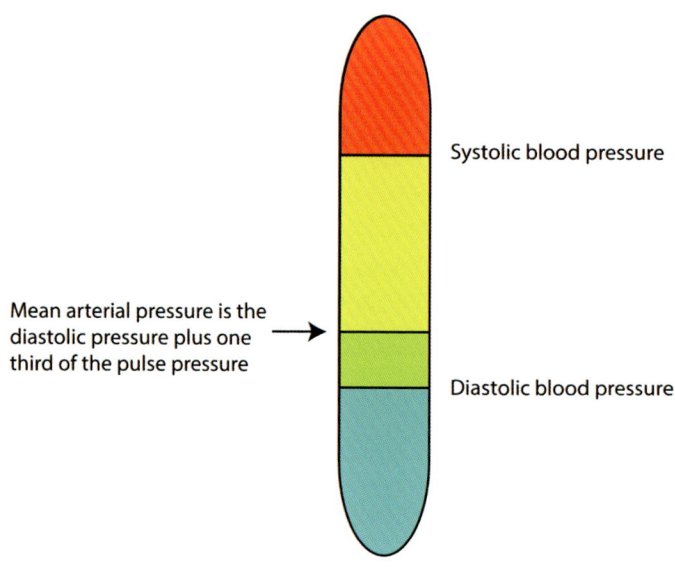

2. **Urine Output > 0.5 ml/kg/hour**

3. **Pulse < 100 beats/minute**

In this case, there was favourable change in pulse, blood pressure and urine output. The urine output (a further 20ml in just 20 minutes) and blood pressure are now both in range with just the first fluid challenge. By no means is this always the case - always reassess and be prepared to repeat! Many patients will benefit from the full 30ml/kg.

HOW DO WE DECIDE WHETHER TO CONTINUE OR STOP FLUID CHALLENGES?

| Dehydrated | Euvolemic | Overloaded |

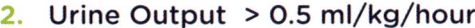

A FIT, YOUNG PERSON HAS A LARGE THERAPEUTIC WINDOW FOR FLUIDS, AND SO A GENEROUS APPROACH TO FLUID USUALLY WORKS.

| Dehydrated | Euvolemic | Overloaded |

A PATIENT WITH A HEART FAILURE HAS A MUCH NARROWER THERAPEUTIC WINDOW FOR FLUIDS, AND SO A MORE CAUTIOUS APPROACH TO FLUID THERAPY IS NEEDED.

Initial presentation

LOW BP, HIGH PULSE, LOW URINE OUTPUT

Repeat fluid challenges until:

TARGET BP, URINE OUTPUT AND PULSE ACHEIVED OR SIGNS OF OVERLOAD OR AT LEAST 30ML/KG GIVEN IN TOTAL

If your initial fluid challenges, to a volume of 30ml per kg body weight, do not restore urine output, heart rate and blood pressure (or if the lactate remains high), this is SEPTIC SHOCK. Septic shock is a critical situation and demands immediate referral to Critical Care.

HOW DO WE DECIDE ABOUT FURTHER FLUIDS AFTER THE FLUID CHALLENGES?

In sepsis without septic shock:

Use the following guides:

1. Clinical scenario
2. Clinical fluid status
3. Observations
4. Markers of end organ perfusion
5. U&Es

The fluid regime for maintenance is not as aggressive as the regime for resuscitation. A typical person needs about 1.5-2.5L of fluid a day. A septic patient who is unable to tolerate oral fluids is likely to need more, to cover additional fluid losses through pyrexia, sweating and the increased respiration rate.

You will need to strongly consider further fluid challenges if the blood pressure, pulse or any markers of end organ hypoperfusion such as urine output and mental status suggest hypovolemia. These challenges are separate from the maintenance fluids.

PATIENTS WITH SEPTIC SHOCK OR LACTATE > 4MMOL/L:

If hypotension is not corrected with fluid challenges, or if lactate is >4 mmol/l, this is septic shock. These patients should be managed in HDU or ITU. Specialists will administer further fluids and commence invasive monitoring and/or drugs acting on the circulation to achieve the following targets within 6 hours:

A. Central venous pressure 8-12 mm Hg
B. Mean arterial pressure (MAP) ≥ 65 mm Hg
C. Urine output ≥ 0.5 mL/kg/hr
D. Central venous (superior vena cava) or mixed venous oxygen saturation 70% or 65%, respectively.

In patients with elevated lactate levels, we should target resuscitation to normalise lactate.

PRACTICAL TIP: "FIRST FLUIDS FAST, SECOND SET SLOWER"

When you see your septic patient, you can deliver three of the Sepsis Six as soon as you have IV access:

1. TAKE BLOOD CULTURES
2. GIVE A STAT IV DOSE OF ANTIBIOTICS
3. GIVE YOUR FIRST FLUIDS FAST

Your usual challenge will be up to 30ml/kg of Hartmann's or Normal Saline 0.9% given in divided boluses as quickly as possible but always within the first hour, although lower volumes (but not lower rates) should be used in those at risk of overload. You might tailor your fluid choice based on the U&Es if these are available, otherwise Hartmann's solution is a sensible choice.

Monitor the response to each fluid challenge, and repeat if MAP < 65, Pulse <100 and/or urine output is less than 0.5ml/kg/hour provided there are no signs of overload.

Stop if there are signs of overload. If you have reached 30ml/kg in total within an hour and the patient remains poorly perfused, or their heart rate, blood pressure, urine output or lactate have not returned to acceptable levels, then refer immediately to Critical Care and tell your senior.

Once the patient has a MAP > 65, a pulse <100 and a urine output > 0.5ml/kg/hour, ensure the patient has regular observations and that further fluids will be prescribed if needed. It is a good idea to write up maintainence fluids e.g. 8 hourly bags of Hartmann's if the patient will not have sufficient oral intake.

These are only guides, and some patients will still need senior review even if you have attained these goals. If the patient 'doesn't look right', trust your instinct!

STEP FIVE: TAKE HAEMOGLOBIN AND LACTATE

Why is lactate a marker of severity in sepsis?

Normally, the body metabolises glucose to produce adenosine triphosphate- the 'energy currency' of the body, known as ATP. The end product of this process (glycolysis) produces another substance called pyruvate. Glycolysis does not require oxygen. The pyruvate is then metabolised with oxygen in the cells' mitochondria to produce more ATP.

If there is a lack of oxygen, pyruvate is instead converted to lactate. This conversion of pyruvate to lactate produces other substances that allow further glycolysis to happen.

Lactate is therefore a marker of anaerobic respiration. Lactate may be elevated when oxygen delivery is inadequate for oxygen demand.

> ### KEY POINT:
> LACTATE IS A MARKER OF ANAEROBIC RESPIRATION. THIS COULD REPRESENT LOCAL OR SYSTEMIC ISCHAEMIA.

A raised arterial lactate is because of one of four types of problems:

1. Insufficient oxygen delivery due to circulatory failure (the 'macrocirculation'), which means a problem with:

$$O_2 \text{ DELIVERY} = O_2 \text{ CONTENT OF BLOOD} \times \text{CARDIAC OUTPUT}$$

2. Insufficient oxygen delivery in the microcirculation (the capillary beds are not working properly)

3. Inability of the tissues to use oxygen (e.g. mitochondrial dysfunction)

4. Excessive oxygen demand e.g. tonic-clonic seizures

Despite optimising oxygen delivery in the macrocirculation through fluid challenges and optimising oxygen content, the lactate may still remain elevated in sepsis. This is partly because in sepsis there may also be microcirculatory derangement

Normally, the microcirculation is regulated by signaling between local cells. These signals help match local tissue oxygen demand with local blood supply. In sepsis, this regulation gets deranged.

The two main issues are:

1. **The flow in some capillaries stops altogether, which leaves tissue perfused by those capillaries hypoxic. This is typically caused by physical obstruction of the capillaries, either by red and white blood cells with reduced deformability or by microthrombi (tiny blood clots) formed by the dysfunctional clotting system**

2. **Increased blood shunting directly from the arterioles (small arteries) to the venules (small veins) without passing through the capillaries, which may cause tissue dependent on those arterioles to become hypoxic.**

A lactate that was high (>4 mmol/L) on presentation but which recovers to normal (<2 mmol/L) following the Sepsis Six and optimization of oxygen delivery suggests the problem was largely in the macrocirculation, which has been fixed for now. This is important, because early correction of oxygen delivery in the macrocirculation may reduce or even stop the development of microcirculation problems.

A lactate that remains high despite optimization of the oxygen delivery is very concerning. This implies that there is also microcirculatory derangement, which needs urgent senior medical advice and likely ITU.

Lactate is useful for three reasons. First, it identifies those patients who have circulatory problems but whose blood pressure is preserved: this is known as 'cryptic shock'. Second, it predicts outcome: a high lactate means there is greater likelihood of a need for Critical Care admission. Third, it helps guide therapy: if it begins to fall with fluid challenges, then the challenges are helping.

WHAT ABOUT Hb?

As we've seen before:

OXYGEN CONTENT/ML =

$$[1.34 \times [Hb] \times (SATURATION/100)]$$
$$+$$
$$0.003 \times PO_2$$

The normal range in the UK for a man is 13.0-18.0 g/dL and for a woman is 11.5-16.5 g/dL (some centres will use g/L, so 130-180 for a man and 115-165 for a woman)

An oxygen saturation of 100% does not necessarily mean the patient has optimal oxygen content in the blood. A reduced [Hb] will decrease the oxygen content of the blood without decreasing the saturation; in other words, a patient who is profoundly anaemic (e.g, haemoglobin of 5.5g/dL) can have a saturation of 100% but will have a very low blood oxygen content.

In general, the factors that will determine the need for red cell transfusion are:

1. The degree of anaemia

An [Hb] < 7g/dL is a commonly used threshold for transfusion. However, the absolute value of the [Hb] alone is not the best marker for guiding transfusion, and the other factors below are at least as significant.

2. The acuteness of the anaemia

The more acute the anaemia (the more quickly it has arisen), the worse it will be tolerated.

3. Co-existing problems with oxygen delivery

In a patient with other problems with oxygen delivery e.g. hypoxia or reduced cardiac output, the anaemia will decompensate them further than an equivalent patient without the hypoxia or reduced cardiac output. For this reason, many centres have higher transfusion targets in patients with cardiac or respiratory disease.

4. Symptoms

A patient who is tachycardic, acidotic, severely short of breath and showing signs of acute heart failure with an [Hb] of 8.1 g/dL is probably more needing of a transfusion than a very comfortable, awake patient with an [Hb] of 6.9 g/dL.

5. Target [Hb]

As a guide, once tissue hypoperfusion has been corrected and in the absence of signficant coronary artery disease, acute hemorrhage, or lactic acidosis, red blood cell transfusion should occur only when hemoglobin decreases to below 7.0 g/dL with a target of 7-9 g/dL.

RISKS OF TRANSFUSION OF BLOOD PRODUCTS

Minor transfusion problems
- FEVER, CHILLS, URTICARIA

Major transfusion problems
- ACUTE HAEMOLYSIS
- DELAYED HAEMOLYSIS
- ANAPHYLAXIS
- TRANSMISSION OF HUMAN IMMUNODEFICIENCY VIRUS, HUMAN T-CELL LYMPHOTROPHIC VIRUS I AND II, HEPATITIS B AND C, CYTOMEGALOVIRUS
- BACTERIAL CONTAMINATION
- GRAFT-VERSUS-HOST DISEASE
- ACUTE LUNG INJURY
- VOLUME OVERLOAD
- HYPOTHERMIA
- IMMUNOMODULATION/ IMMUNOSUPPRESSION

STEP SIX: MONITOR URINE OUTPUT AND FLUID BALANCE (+/– CATHETERISE)

URINE OUTPUT

In the early stages, urine output **is key.**

Most people will present for the first time with sepsis in primary care, on the ward or in the Emergency Department or Medical/ Surgical Admissions Unit, not in Intensive Care. This means that there will be little or no access to cardiac output monitoring.

The perfusion of tissues is dependent upon blood pressure (the force needed to overcome resistance- if BP is too low, the cells at the peripheries will not receive blood flow) and blood flow, which is determined by cardiac output.

A patient with a blood pressure of 80/40, and a cardiac output of 8 litres per minute, is in better shape than a patient with a blood pressure of 150/100 and a cardiac output of 0.5 litres per minute

In healthcare, we have become over-reliant on blood pressure, probably because it's easier to measure. For patients with sepsis, it is critical to have another window on the circulation- and urine output provides this.

Urine output (at least in health) is relatively independent of blood pressure due to a process known as autoregulation, although the effect of this diminishes in critical illness. As the diagram shows, blood flow through the kidneys remains fairly constant over a range of blood pressure:

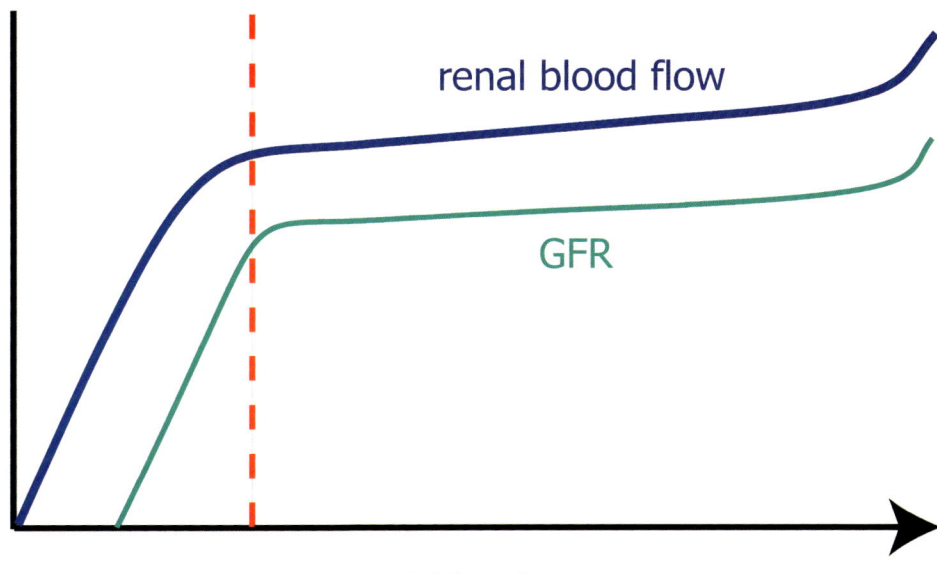

autoregulation fails at blood pressures to the left of this line

renal blood flow

GFR

arterial blood pressure

However, the kidneys cannot autoregulate well for changes in blood flow. The relationship here is quite linear- as blood flow to the kidneys falls, so does glomerular filtration rate and therefore urine output.

The urine output is an excellent window on the circulation. As blood flow (cardiac output) falls, so does urine output. This is essential in guiding further fluid challenges, and may identify a problem with the circulation before the blood pressure begins to fall.

FLUID BALANCE

Can't we just compare the inputs and the outputs to decide about fluid balance?

The fluid balance chart does not take into account insensible losses and gains.

Insensible losses/gains are different from other losses because they are losses of free water only, not water and solute.

INSENSIBLE LOSSES

Skin: about 400-500ml/day. Increased in pyrexia and sweating.

Respiratory: about 400-500ml/day. Increased in with hyperventilation. Decreased with humidified inspired air/oxygen.

INSENSIBLE GAIN

Metabolism: about 400ml/day.

It may seem that the input should be about 400ml greater than the output in a 'typical' fluid balance chart. However, the insensible losses are impossible to measure, and what is going on in each patient is so variable that it is meaningless to target a particular number of mls to cover this theoretical difference based on the average relatively well patient.

Instead, we should be guided by:

1. Clinical scenario
2. Clinical assessment of fluid status
3. Observations
4. Markers of end organ perfusion and hydration (mucous membranes, capillary refill, mental status, urine output, lactate and central venous saturations)
5. U&Es

The numbers given by daily requirements are just guides; what you actually prescribe is determined by these factors.

SO WHAT IS THE POINT OF A FLUID BALANCE CHART?

If input >> output, then one of four scenarios is usually happening:

1. The patient is dehydrated, and whatever oral/
   IV fluids have been given are well needed
2. The patient is getting overloaded with excessive fluids
3. There is a renal/endocrine problem with the production of urine
4. There is a urological problem with the outflow of urine

If output >> input, then one of five scenarios is usually happening:

1. The patient is becoming rapidly dehydrated, with
   insufficient fluid to replace losses
2. The patient is overloaded, and is appropriately offloading fluid
3. Inappropriate use of diuretic
4. There is a polyuric renal problem
5. Recovery from pre-renal Acute Kidney Injury (requires observation only)

PRACTICAL TIP: SO EASILY DONE...
DON'T FORGET TO START A FLUID BALANCE CHART ONCE YOU HAVE PUT THE CATHETER IN!

SEPSIS. SPOT IT. TREAT IT. BEAT IT.

FURTHER READING

TRZECIAK S, CHANSKY ME, DELLINGER PR ET AL. OPERATIONALIZING THE USE OF
SERUM LACTATE MEASUREMENT FOR IDENTIFYING HIGH RISK OF DEATH IN A CLINICAL PRACTICE
ALGORITHM FOR SUSPECTED SEVERE SEPSIS. ACAD EMERG MED 2006; 13: 150-1

DANIELS R, NUTBEAM T, MCNAMARA G, GALVIN C. THE SEPSIS SIX AND THE
SEVERE SEPSIS RESUSCITATION BUNDLE: A PROSPECTIVE OBSERVATIONAL
COHORT STUDY. EMERG MED J 2010; DOI:10.1136/EMJ.2010.095067

BRITISH THORACIC SOCIETY EMERGENCY OXYGEN GROUP. GUIDELINE FOR EMERGENCY
OXYGEN USE IN ADULT PATIENTS. THORAX 2008; 63 (SUPPL VI): 1-81

COMMON PRESENTATIONS OF SEPSIS

INTRODUCTION

Severe sepsis has an associated mortality of around 30-35%, yet only one out of every five patients with sepsis receives care in accordance with international guidelines. Sepsis should be seen as a medical emergency. A patient with severe sepsis has a higher chance of dying than a patient suffering a stroke or heart attack. Simple interventions should be initiated promptly. These include the Sepsis Six. Mortality can be halved simply by giving these simple measures, including intravenous antibiotics and intravenous fluids, promptly. Early treatment not only improves patient outcomes but has a huge economic benefit too.

The clinical signs and symptoms of early sepsis are often vague, subtle or non-specific; for instance tachycardia or fever. This makes it difficult to diagnose as early signs can often be missed by healthcare providers. Few doctors can describe the definition of sepsis accurately, so it is no surprise that sepsis can be difficult to manage. The lack of awareness surrounding this condition contributes to poor patient outcomes. Early screening and early and aggressive treatment in patients presenting with sepsis is key in improving patient outcomes.

This chapter aims to increase your knowledge surrounding common presentations of sepsis, and how to recognise and treat this condition appropriately.

OBJECTIVES:

By the end of this chapter you should

1. Be aware of some of the common presentations of sepsis

2. Be familiar with the initial assessment and management of a septic patient

3. Be aware of common pitfalls in the recognition and treatment of sepsis

4. Be aware of atypical presentations of sepsis and special patient groups (i.e. the septic elderly patient)

CASE STUDY

The death of Christopher Reeve, the actor who played Superman in 2004, was attributed to heart failure secondary to sepsis. Although the exact cause will never be known as there was no autopsy, he was suffering with a number of pressure sores at the time. This may have been the source of his sepsis which led to cardiovascular collapse and eventually resulted in his death.

Mr Reeves's sepsis went unrecognised until he developed cardiovascular compromise. He was rushed to hospital when he suffered a cardiac arrest, but by then it was too late. Perhaps if the early signs of sepsis had been recognised at the start, then the outcome would have been different.

RECOGNITION OF SEPSIS

We have discussed the use of a sepsis screening tool to identify those patients with severe sepsis in a previous chapter. This screening tool applies to all patients across a given hospital, and should be used in conjunction with clinical skills and with existing observations and 'track-and-trigger' systems such as Modified or National Early Warning Scores (MEWS) and Patient at Risk Scores (PARS).

In all cases, the key to successful early recognition of patients, and therefore to completion of the Sepsis Six and Septic Shock Bundle (see module on advanced resuscitation), is a high index of suspicion. For example, patients with pneumonia comprise the largest group of patients with severe sepsis, so all patients with pneumonia must have the screening tool applied on admission and at any point of deterioration. In patients presenting in a collapsed state or with a general deterioration, severe sepsis must be considered in the differential diagnosis along with conditions such as stroke, metabolic disorders and cardiac failure.

In any patient in whom severe sepsis is identified, a thorough search for the source of sepsis will be required. This may require consultation with colleagues in radiology and surgery. While the search for the source is on-going, empiric broad spectrum antibiotics to cover any likely pathogens must be initiated. If a source amenable to drainage is found, this should be performed without delay, and certainly within 12 hours following the onset of sepsis.

It must be remembered that patients with sepsis may present when they deteriorate during treatment for an unrelated condition, or if they fail to improve as expected. In other words, patients may develop sepsis after they arrive in hospital, and we must take care not to be 'blinkered' to the original diagnosis. This phenomenon is also known as a loss of situational awareness- a 'step back' to look at the big picture can often prevent this.

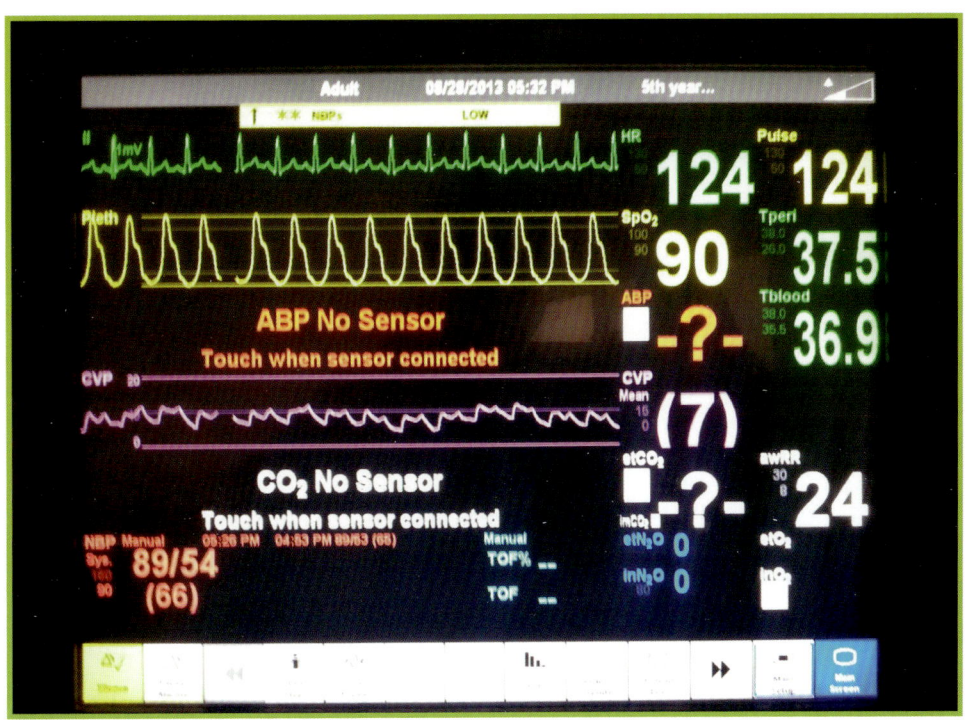

CASE STUDY

For this case put yourself in the patient's position and imagine what it would be like if you came into the Emergency Department (ED) in the following scenario:

You have been feeling feverish and unwell for a few days, and you have been complaining of urinary frequency and urgency associated with foul smelling urine. Today you feel more unwell and you think the fever is worse.

17.00: Arrival in ED: Your observations are: RR 20, sats 95%, HR 110bpm, BP 110/86 mmHg, temp 38.8°C, U/O 35ml/hour

Investigations include: WCC 16 x 10^9/l, plt 358 x 10^9/l, Hb 11.5g/dL, glucose 8.0mmol/l, urea 6mmol/l, creatinine 95mmol/l, lactate 3.5mmol/l

You are diagnosed with pyelonephritis and admitted under the medical team. You are written up for IV antibiotics and IV Hartmann's is started at 100ml/hr.

You are transferred to the medical ward before these are administered. On the ward, no-one thinks to check for any prescriptions until the next routine drug round at 20:00.

20.30: Feeling worse Observations: RR 26, Sats 88% FiO_2 0.5, HR 115bpm, BP 88/58 mmHg, temp 38.9°C, U/O 10ml/hour

Critical Care Outreach assessment: Lactate 5.6mmol/l, blood gas (metabolic acidosis): pH 7.25, pO_2 7.5 kPa, pCO_2 3.8kPa, HCO3- 26mmol/l

A decision is made to transfer you to intensive care for management of your severe sepsis. You now have a mortality risk of up to 70% with three organ failure.

This is an example of poor early management of severe sepsis. On arrival in the Emergency Department, although this patient's blood pressure was normal, her heart rate and lactate were suggestive of hypoperfusion of major organs. Fluid resuscitation should have been more aggressive, and she should have been re-assessed regularly. Similarly, writing an antibiotic up (especially without a 'stat' dose) typically results in delays of several hours unless the urgency is communicated well. This patient should have been fluid resuscitated, her antibiotic given, and been re-assessed before she left the ED. Like an acute myocardial infarction, this condition is time sensitive. The longer you go without treatment, the longer your organs will go without oxygen. Think of it as 'time to organs'. Remember to get senior help early and initiate treatment promptly.

The following conditions are listed to aid diagnosis in some of the more common presentations. A background history if available will be vital to establish the possible sources of sepsis, or a predisposition to particular infections– for instance septic arthritis in a patient with rheumatoid arthritis.

Treatment for severe sepsis in these patients will not differ from any other. Following immediate assessment using ABCDE, the Sepsis Six are the first priority toward completing the Surviving Sepsis Campaign's Severe Sepsis Bundle. Some guidance as to the suggested antimicrobial strategy is given, but it is emphasised that this is no substitute for local knowledge and local microbiology guidelines.

In all of these conditions, it is assumed that basic tests such as full blood count, urea and electrolytes, blood sugar, liver function tests, coagulation screen and arterial blood gases (including lactate level) will have been done.

PNEUMONIA

As we have discussed, this condition accounts for the largest proportion of patients presenting with severe sepsis. The patient may present with a cough, purulent sputum, pleuritic pain (worse on deep inspiration) or haemoptysis (coughing up blood). These features are non-specific for pneumonia and each could occur in other conditions, for instance in pulmonary embolus.

The typical history is one of a progressive cough and dyspnoea (difficulty with breathing) over a short period. 'Atypical' pneumonias (caused by less common microbes such as Legionella pneumonia) can present in a more subtle way, commonly with a vague flu-like illness or a headache with a dry cough, sometimes developing over weeks rather than days.

Patients will often be tachypnoeic (respiratory rates may be over 40 per minute in severe cases) and breathing may be noisy, sometimes with audible 'rattles' from the end of the bed. If severe sepsis has already developed, systemic signs as discussed in previous chapters may be present.

If skilled to examine the chest, signs of consolidation may be noted. These include dullness of the chest to percussion, added sounds such as crackles and bronchial breathing, and reduced air entry over the affected part of the chest.

It is worth remembering that we lose a large amount of fluid through respiration. Particularly if a patient has been breathing un-humidified (dry) oxygen-enriched air for a period of time, dehydration can be a prominent feature of pneumonia. The reason for this is that fluid from the patient's airways evaporates to moisten the dry inhaled air, and is replaced from the extracellular fluid. This is one form of insensible loss- a fluid shift which we are unable to measure.

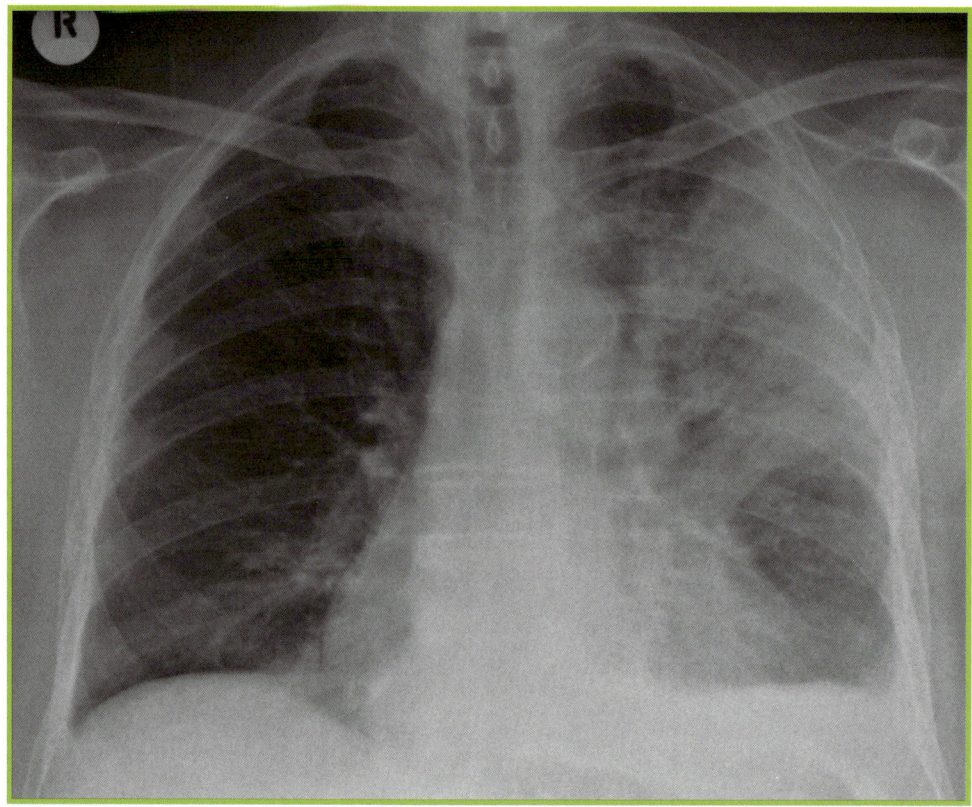

WITH PERMISSION FROM RADIOLOGYMASTERCLASS.CO.UK

Investigations to confirm the diagnosis and look for the underlying cause include a CXR, whilst cultures of sputum and blood should be sent. **Don't wait for a chest X ray to confirm pneumonia before starting treatment if severe sepsis is present.** If an atypical organism is likely then serology for organisms such as Legionella or Mycoplasma should be requested, along with urine samples to look for the relevant antigens- some organisations prefer to screen for these routinely, and some screen routinely for the Human Immunodeficiency Virus (HIV) in cases of severe community-acquired pneumonia. It is always best to liaise with microbiology if you suspect an atypical pneumonia. Occasionally an immunocompromised patient may have an organism such as Pneumocystis carinii, which may require bronchial lavage to get a confirmed diagnosis. If tuberculosis is suspected then early morning sputum specimens are useful, and occasionally a gastric aspirate may be required to catch sputum that has been swallowed.

Patients should be assessed serially for signs of decompensation or fatigue. Arterial blood gases are useful in this regard. The patient will commonly present with near-normal levels of arterial oxygen, which may gradually drop as the condition progresses. The onset of hypercapnia (a high level of carbon dioxide), particularly if worsening, mandates immediate referral to Critical Care.

Antibiotics should be tailored to the source. Community acquired pneumonia is likely to be streptococcal (caused by Streptococcus pneumoniae) or due to Haemophilus influenzae, so intravenous benzylpenicillin and levofloxacin or clarithromycin are a good choice. Erythromycin is a suitable alternative in penicillin allergic patients.

If aspiration pneumonia is likely, then anaerobic organisms can be covered by adding metronidazole. It is not appropriate to start antibiotics 'just in case' in patients with suspected aspiration unless a pneumonia is suspected. Healthcare-associated infections may require a broad spectrum cephalosporin or an anti-pseudomonal penicillin such as piperacillin with tazobactam ('Tazocin'®). If the patient is a resident in a long-term care facility, has had recent hospitalization or is known to be colonized with MRSA, linezolid should be considered as vancomycin penetrates lung tissue poorly.

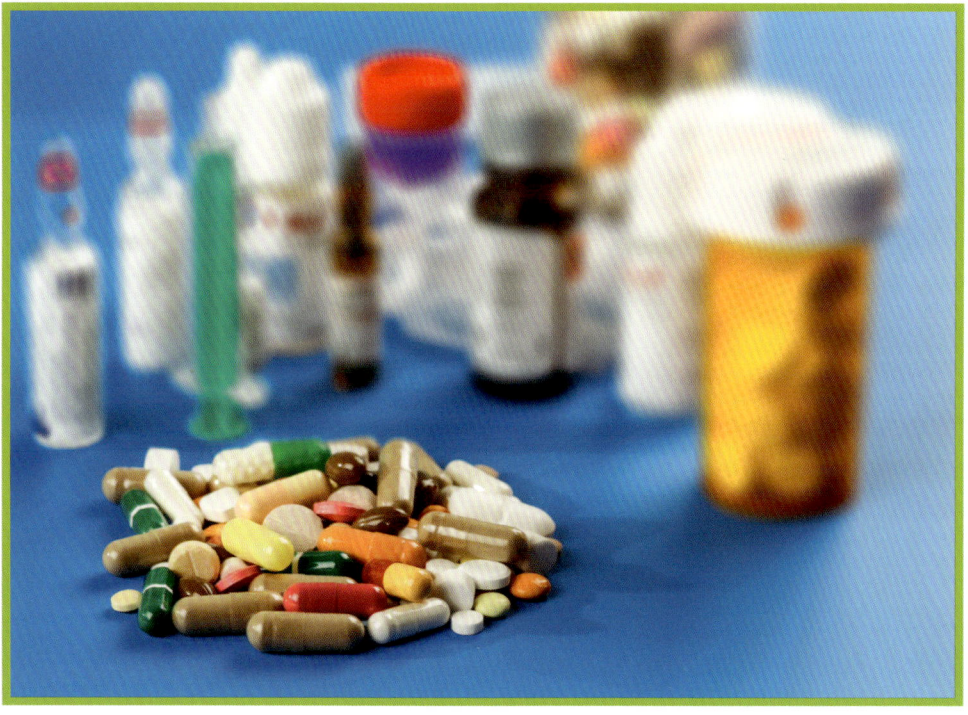

URINARY TRACT SEPSIS

Symptoms can include dysuria (pain on passing urine), frequency, loin pain, and haematuria (blood in urine). The patient may complain of offensive smelling urine. Less commonly, the patient may present in renal failure with non-specific symptoms such as nausea or anorexia. Clinical examination may reveal loin pain, lower abdominal tenderness or distension.

A positive urine dipstick in the absence of symptoms is not a reason to start an antibiotic

Sending urine and blood cultures will aid the diagnosis. A renal ultrasound would be a good initial investigation to look for an underlying cause such as pyelonephritis or renal tract obstruction due to stones. Other imaging such as CT or contrast studies may be required. It is advisable to liaise with colleagues in urology and radiology if a structural abnormality is likely.

Common organisms causing renal tract sepsis are gram-negative bacteria such as E. coli and Klebsiella, so a stat dose of gentamicin followed by levofloxacin until a definite organism is identified are reasonable choices. Resistant ESBL-producing organisms are becoming more prevalent, and around one-third of E.coli in some regions are now resistant to co-amoxiclav. So again it is important to take advice from microbiology.

INTRA-ABDOMINAL SEPSIS

Intra-abdominal sepsis is the second commonest cause of severe sepsis in the general population. A detailed history is essential in determining the likely source of the patient's sepsis. Abdominal examination is important and should include a PR and perianal examination to exclude a perianal abscess. Non-specific symptoms can be a sign that the patient is acutely unwell, such as fever, warm skin from vasodilation or altered mental state. More specific symptoms include abdominal pain. This can be generalised, for instance in generalised peritonitis or localised, for example, in acute appendicitis or cholecystitis. Other associated symptoms may include nausea, vomiting diarrhoea or absolute constipation (no passage of flatus or faeces). Peritonism is classically seen as a tense, rigid abdomen with excruciating pain on palpation- the patient will 'guard' against this by tensing their abdominal muscles. They may also show rebound tenderness, where taking the palpating hand away suddenly causes a pain which is just as severe. However, peritonitis can be present without these signs so beware being falsely reassured. Remember to keep an open mind as abdominal findings can be subtle or absent, and there are many conditions which may mimic intra-abdominal sepsis such as acute pancreatitis or ischaemic bowel. A gynaecological cause for abdominal pain in a female patient should be excluded, for instance a pelvic abscess, ruptured ectopic or torted ovarian cyst. Be guided by your history and clinical findings, and do not forget to do a pregnancy test and seek gynaecological advice.

Patients with intra-abdominal sepsis can deteriorate quickly and require rapid assessment, resuscitation and, if there is thought to be a perforated viscus or anastomotic leak, transfer to a high dependency or intensive care unit 'for resuscitation prior to corrective surgery.

In a patient who has undergone abdominal surgery, a new onset of atrial fibrillation in the absence of grossly abnormal electrolytes is a common sign of developing sepsis.

A senior surgical opinion should be sought at the earliest opportunity as surgical intervention may be needed to resolve the infection. The procedure will obviously depend on the suspected source of infection. Non-operative management of intra-abdominal sepsis can include drainage (for example of an abscess) under radiological guidance.

There are more bacteria within the gut than there are cells in the rest of the body. Abdominal sepsis arising from the gastrointestinal tract is nearly always due to gram-negative organisms, which can enter the bloodstream after migrating from the gut.

BILIARY/GALLBLADDER SEPSIS (CHOLANGITIS/CHOLECYSTITIS)

Abdominal pain in the right upper quadrant is indicative of biliary tract aetiology. Other symptoms can include fever, jaundice or dark urine and pale stools. Biliary sepsis is a frequently missed diagnosis, and elderly patients and diabetics often present atypically. To spot it requires a high index of suspicion in patients without more immediately obvious sources of severe sepsis.

Blood cultures may grow gram-negative organisms. The mainstay of treatment is antibiotic therapy, for instance with intravenous amoxicillin, gentamicin and metronidazole, however local advice must be sought. Drainage of the biliary tree is of equal priority.

An ultrasound of the biliary tract is helpful in identifying or excluding gall stones in the common bile duct, which may be amenable to endoscopic removal. An ERCP may be required to remove common duct stones, so it is important to take advice from the gastroenterology team. In acute cholecystitis a surgical opinion should be sought regarding a cholecystectomy.

ACUTE APPENDICITIS

Appendicitis is one of the commonest surgical emergencies. It occurs typically in the younger population and classically presents with a history of anorexia and umbilical pain which localises to the right iliac fossa (RIF). Examination may reveal tenderness and localised guarding in this area. The patient may be systemically unwell with fever and tachycardia, however it is a clinical diagnosis as there is no single symptom or test to accurately confirm the diagnosis. Antibiotics have an important role in treatment and should cover both aerobic and anaerobic organisms. Appendicectomy is the definitive treatment.

CASE STUDY

A 46 year old male weighing 85kg presents to the Emergency Department with a five day history of severe abdominal pain and constipation. He is complaining of left sided lower abdominal pain. On examination his abdomen is distended and he is tender over his left lower quadrant, with rebound tenderness. Bowel sounds are reduced, and there is hard stool on PR examination.

He has a PMH of controlled hypertension, and takes anti-hypertensives.

Observations are: RR 18, sats 96%, HR 105 bpm, BP 105/82mmHg, temp 39.0°C, U/O 30ml/hour

Investigations show: WCC 17 x 10^9/l plt 254 x 10^9/l, Hb 13.0g/dL, glucose 7.2mmol/l, urea 4.6mmol/l, creatinine 105mmol/l, lactate 2.1mmol/l

WHAT IS THE LIKELY DIAGNOSIS?

DOES HE MEET THE CRITERIA FOR SEPSIS/SEVERE SEPSIS?

WHAT WILL YOUR INITIAL MANAGEMENT BE?

DIVERTICULITIS

Diverticula are small outpouchings of the bowel wall which become inflamed (diverticulitis) and can perforate. Left lower quadrant pain in the commonest presentation for this condition, other symptoms can include nausea, vomiting and altered bowel habit. The diagnosis can be made clinically but a CT scan of the abdomen is the preferred method to confirm the diagnosis. Seek a surgical opinion to decide whether the patient can be managed conservatively, or will need surgical intervention. Patients will require antibiotics. Amoxycillin, gentamicin and metronidazole would be a suitable initial regime, however local microbiology advice should be sought.

CASE STUDY ANSWERS

THIS PATIENT HAS PRESENTED WITH AN ACUTE ABDOMEN. HIS CONSTIPATION AND ABDOMINAL DISTENSION ARE IN KEEPING WITH INTESTINAL OBSTRUCTION, WHILE HIS SEVERE PAIN AND HIGH TEMPERATURE AND WHITE CELL COUNT SUGGEST AN INFECTIVE SOURCE E.G. A PERFORATED VISCUS. CAUSES COULD INCLUDE A CARCINOMA CAUSING OBSTRUCTION AND SECONDARY PERFORATION, A PERFORATED DIVERTICULUM OR ADHESIONS IN A PATIENT WHO HAS PREVIOUSLY UNDERGONE SURGERY.

THIS PATIENT MEETS THE CRITERIA FOR SEVERE SEPSIS. HE HAS A PROBABLE INFECTIVE SOURCE, WITH THE PRESENCE OF 3 SIRS CRITERIA. HE HAS DECREASED URINE OUTPUT, ELEVATED LACTATE, AND HYPOTENSION RELATIVE TO HIS USUAL HYPERTENSION, EACH OF WHICH MEET CRITERIA FOR SEVERE SEPSIS.

MANAGEMENT WILL FOLLOW THE ABCDE APPROACH AND IMPLEMENTATION OF THE SEPSIS SIX. AN ERECT CXR IS HELPFUL TO LOOK FOR AIR UNDER THE DIAPHRAGM, A SIGN OF A PERFORATED VISCUS, AND AN ABDOMINAL CT SHOULD BE CONSIDERED. EARLY SURGICAL REVIEW IS NEEDED AS THIS PATIENT WILL LIKELY NEED TO GO TO THEATRE. IF HIS CIRCULATORY FUNCTION FAILS TO IMPROVE FOLLOWING DELIVERY OF THE SEPSIS SIX, HE WILL REQUIRE REFERRAL TO CRITICAL CARE.

SOFT TISSUE INFECTION

Cellulitis

There is likely to be tenderness, pain and swelling of the affected area possibly following injury or an insect bite, but there may be no obvious precipitant. Diabetic patients are more prone to cellulitis, so it is important to check for a history of diabetes and perform blood glucose measurement in case of undiagnosed diabetes: you might spot a presentation diabetic keto-acidosis! Cellulitis usually presents with rapidly spreading erythema, blistering, or even skin necrosis. The skin will feel hot. In extreme cases it is important to examine for circulatory or neural compromise due to pressure on vessels and nerves from the tense swelling, called "compartment syndrome". It may be necessary to liaise with plastic, orthopaedic or general surgeons if the swelling is causing compartment syndrome. Blood and wound swab culture will hopefully identify an organism (Staphylococci and Streptococci most commonly, but many are polymicrobial). Intravenous benzylpenicillin and flucloxacillin provide adequate cover for sensitive Staphylococci and Streptococci and are a suitable initial choice.

Beware of rapidly spreading cellulitis, or pain disproportionate to the findings. This may be necrotizing fasciitis, a rare surgical emergency, which spreads along fascial planes with destruction of underlying tissue. It is commonly associated with Group A beta-haemolytic streptococci. This group of organisms release exotoxins which worsen the inflammatory response. It has a high associated mortality and requires rapid and extensive debridement of the affected area in theatre as an emergency.

Wound infection

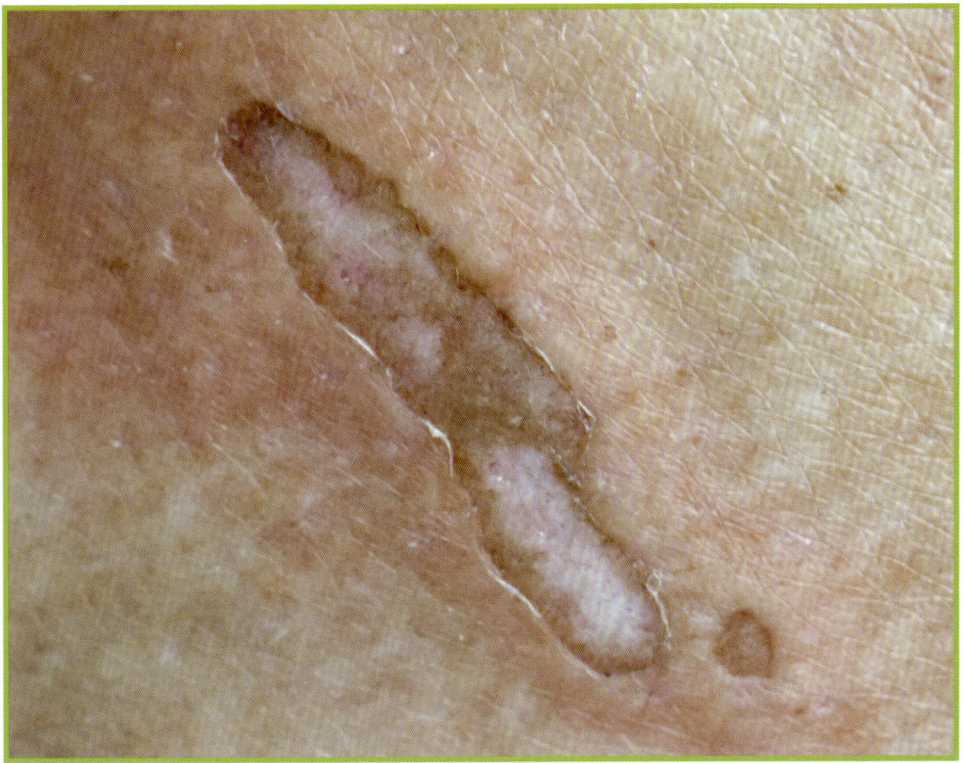

A post-operative wound infection is recognised by pain, erythema, a purulent discharge or heat around the incision. Poor healing may be the first marker of a lower grade infection. Although wound infections start as localised infections, they do form part of the group of soft tissue infections responsible for 5-10% of all causes of severe sepsis. Post-operative wounds should be inspected daily and if there is evidence of discharge the clips or sutures should be removed and the potential space opened up using a gloved finger. Antibiotics are not needed unless a patient is immunosuppressed or there is evidence of surrounding cellulitis. Consideration should be given to the presence of a deeper infection- for example, an infected joint prosthesies or leaking abdominal anastomosis.

MENINGITIS

CASE STUDY

A 40 year old woman weighing 60kg presents to your Emergency Department with a severe headache. She complains of photophobia, and she has not experienced such a severe headache before.

Observations are: RR22, sats 95%, HR 108 bpm, BP 102/76mmHg, temp 38.9°C, U/O 40ml/hour

Investigations show: WCC 22 x 10^9/l plt 388 x 10^9/l, Hb 12.0g/dL, glucose 9.0mmol/l, urea 5mmol/l, creatinine 76µmol/l, lactate 2.5mmol/l

WHAT IS THE MOST LIKELY DIAGNOSIS?

HOW WOULD YOU DEFINE HER CONDITION USING THE CRITERIA FOR SEPSIS AND SEVERE SEPSIS?

WHAT IS THE MOST APPROPRIATE IMMEDIATE MANAGEMENT?

It is important to differentiate between meningitis (inflammation of the meninges, usually due to infection) and meningococcal septicaemia or sepsis. Each can exist without the other. Meningococcal sepsis, if present, carries a far worse prognosis than meningitis alone.

Symptoms of meningitis include headache, photophobia, vomiting, a stiff neck, or drowsiness. Symptoms of meningococcal sepsis include some of the above- vomiting and drowsiness- plus rigors, cold hands and feet sometimes with severe pain, confusion and myalgia (muscle pain). Awareness campaigns have raised the knowledge of these symptoms amongst the general public but they can still progress very rapidly in a previously well patient. Those who have dealt with these patients will be only too aware of the alarming rate at which a previously healthy person can deteriorate to severe multi-organ failure.

The incidence of meningitis has, thankfully, reduced dramatically due to vaccination programmes. However, for the individual patient we must not let our guard down and retain a high index of suspicion.

Signs of meningitis include neck rigidity, a decreased level of consciousness or occasionally focal neurological signs. Worsening neurological signs may indicate the development of cerebral oedema or hydrocephalus (raised pressure in the cranial cavity due to obstruction of cerebrospinal fluid flow).

If meningococcal sepsis is present, a typical purpuric (like small bruises) rash may be noted, and frequently signs of circulatory failure- shock, cold and mottled peripheries, low urine output and reduced conscious level.

Blood cultures should be performed immediately (along with other baseline blood tests). A lumbar puncture should be done if possible to culture organisms and check CSF protein level, white cell count and glucose level. If there is doubt about the diagnosis (for instance a subarachnoid haemorrhage may have some similar clinical features) or there is any suspicion of raised intracranial pressure then a CT head may be required.

It is vital not to delay treatment. Intravenous antibiotics with activity against the Meningococcus (Neisseria meningitidis) such as cefotaxime/ceftriaxone should be given immediately. If blood cultures are likely to cause delays and this cannot be avoided, then antibiotics should take priority.

The presence of a meningococcal rash denotes meningococcal septicaemia. This is a medical emergency and demands the highest level of skill and experience available. It is inappropriate for a junior to manage such cases alone.

If you see a purpuric rash, get senior help immediately

CASE STUDY ANSWERS

THIS LADY ALMOST CERTAINLY HAS MENINGITIS. SHE HAS A SOURCE OF INFECTION ASSOCIATED WITH FOUR SIRS CRITERIA (WCC > 12X10^9/L, TEMP > 38.3 °C, RR > 20/MIN, HR > 90/MIN) IN KEEPING WITH SEPSIS. HER LACTATE OF 2.5MMOL/L QUALIFIES HER AS SEVERE SEPSIS AT THIS POINT.

IMMEDIATE MANAGEMENT WOULD FOLLOW AN ABCDE APPROACH, AND IMPLEMENTATION OF THE SEPSIS SIX. COMMENCE HIGH FLOW OXYGEN; TAKE CULTURES FOR BLOOD AND CSF (TIME PERMITTING BUT DO NOT DELAY ANTIBIOTIC TREATMENT), START IV ANTIBIOTICS AND IV FLUIDS. MONITOR HOURLY U/O AND CALL FOR SENIOR HELP WITH REPEATED RE-ASSESSMENT- THIS LADY MAY DETERIORATE WITHIN MINUTES.

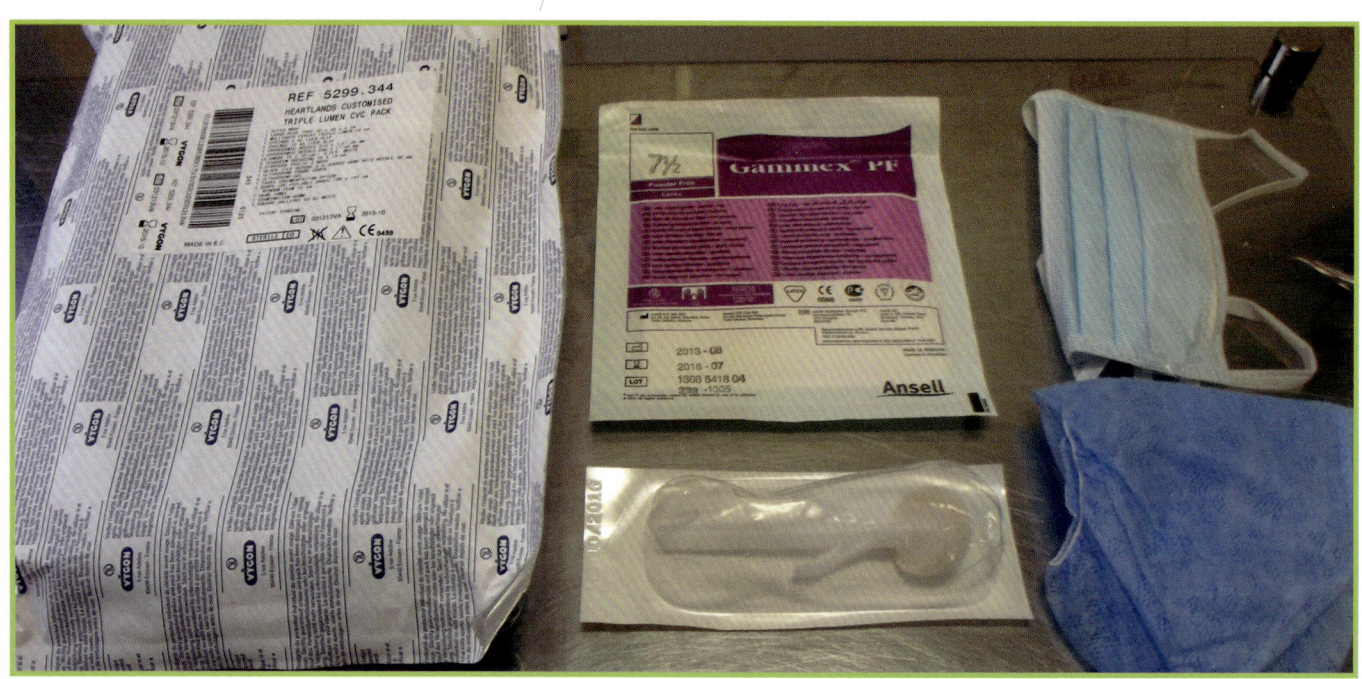

LINE SEPSIS

Sepsis can by associated with the direct introduction of microbes into the blood stream through insertion of lines. Inspect any intravenous (IV) or intra-arterial lines for signs of sepsis and, if there is erythema or swelling around a line, the line should be removed and the tip cultured.

Central IV lines are the most commonly associated with bacteraemia, be suspicious of a central line in place for over a week. Peripheral venous lines are less commonly involved, particularly since the introduction of high impact care bundles for their insertion and management, and arterial lines even less so. Do not forget to check the site of the urethral catheter and the epidural if present.

SEPTIC ARTHRITIS

Symptoms include severe pain (particularly on movement) of an infected joint, swelling and often a history of arthritis. It is important to ask about trauma or recent instrumentation to the joint such as arthroscopic surgery. Usually the joint will be hot, swollen, red and extremely tender, with a limited range of movement.

Joint aspiration is vital to establish the diagnosis and identify the causative organism. Any aspirate should be sent for culture and microscopy. Blood cultures should also be sent. X-rays or other imaging will be required to establish the extent of any joint destruction.

Any antibiotic therapy must cover Staphylococci and achieve good joint penetration – intravenous benzylpenicillin and flucloxacillin being a good initial choice. It is important to liaise with orthopaedic surgeons and/or rheumatologists. In many cases a joint washout by arthroscopy is warranted, and should be completed within the first 12 hours. In the recovery phase physiotherapy will be essential to regain joint function.

ENDOCARDITIS

This is not a common condition to present acutely as severe sepsis, but should be considered if a septic patient has no other obvious source of infection, and in particular if there is a history of heart valve disease or rheumatic fever in childhood. Symptoms include dyspnoea, weight loss, and swinging fevers. Heart murmurs may be significant, particularly if they are new or changing. Remember, however, that a lot of healthy people will have trivial murmurs.

Splinter haemorrhages on the nails may be a feature (but are often innocent due to finger trauma, particularly if the patient has a manual occupation). In sub-acute endocarditis splenomegaly may occur. The patient can appear cachectic, and may be mistakenly thought to have a malignancy. They may have signs of heart failure such as raised jugular venous pressure, peripheral oedema and pulmonary congestion.

Bacterial endocarditis is another condition that may be missed when a patient develops severe sepsis for the first time in hospital, particularly on Critical Care. The use of central venous catheters provides microorganisms with a direct route to the heart. The key to spotting endocarditis lies in a high index of suspicion in patients who have severe sepsis of unknown cause.

Multiple sets of blood cultures from different sites are mandatory. These may take several days to grow an organism. An echocardiogram should be requested to look for vegetations, but absence of these does not exclude the diagnosis. Trans-oesophageal echocardiography (TOE) may be necessary.

It is mandatory to involve Cardiology early, as the patient may deteriorate and may require urgent valve replacement surgery. It is also important to link with microbiology but initially intravenous benzylpenicillin or amoxicillin together with gentamicin would be a reasonable choice. Again, staphylococci are frequent culprits, and vancomycin can be considered. Long durations of antibiotic treatments are often necessary.

- Consider sepsis when a patient being treated for another condition suddenly deteriorates.

- Sepsis may be iatrogenic (IV cannula insertion, catheter change, post procedure such as ERCP). In this case remove the source whenever possible.

- Immunocompromised patients (those on chemotherapy, steroids, patients with AIDS etc.) can develop sepsis rapidly and may not always have localising signs – urgent antibiotic therapy is required before waiting for test results.

- Partially treated infections may relapse and may then yield resistant organisms (bone, joint and heart infections require prolonged courses).

- Hidden sources of sepsis include pressure sores and intra-abdominal sepsis (e.g. spontaneous bacterial peritonitis common in alcoholics). Remember, a medical patient may develop an acute abdomen, while a surgical patient may develop pneumonia post-operatively.

- Has the patient travelled abroad? Think malaria, TB, dysentery.

- Multi resistant organisms may account for why a patient is not improving.

SPECIAL PATIENT GROUPS

THE IMMUNOCOMPROMISED PATIENT

- This group includes haematology cancer patients and post-chemotherapy patients. These groups are beyond the remit of this chapter, but will demand the early involvement of specialist care at the highest level.

- Existing protocols for neutropenic sepsis should be adhered to, and supplemented if necessary with Early Goal-Directed Therapy.

THE ELDERLY PATIENT

- The elderly patient presents a unique set of problems. They may present non-specifically, for example with hypotension and collapse, or with confusion. The latter is sometimes mis-attributed to a simple urinary tract in this group of patients, but always warrants an open mind and full investigation.

- The elderly may not mount an effective immune response. Their white cell count may not always be markedly raised, leading to confusion in establishing the diagnosis.

- Elderly patients have lower physiological reserves in terms of their cardiovascular and respiratory systems. They tend to develop shock much earlier than younger patients, and are at high risk therefore of multi-organ failure and death. Tachycardia is often not marked.

- Pre-existing malnourishment may make an elderly patient slower to recover. Other co-morbidities, such as diabetes and heart failure are also more common, and may impede recovery.

THE PREGNANT PATIENT

- The commonest causes of sepsis in pregnancy are urosepsis, thought to be related to mechanical ureteric obstruction from the gravid uterus, and genital tract sepsis. Specific guidance on managing sepsis in the pregnancy and the puerperium are available from the Royal College of Obstetricians and Gynaecologists' Green Top series.

- Sepsis is the biggest direct cause of maternal death. A pregnant patient or a new mum (particularly if she has had instrumentation or surgical assistance) with suspected sepsis should always be seen by a senior immediately.

- An acute abdomen may be difficult to diagnose in a pregnant patient, and they can often present atypically.

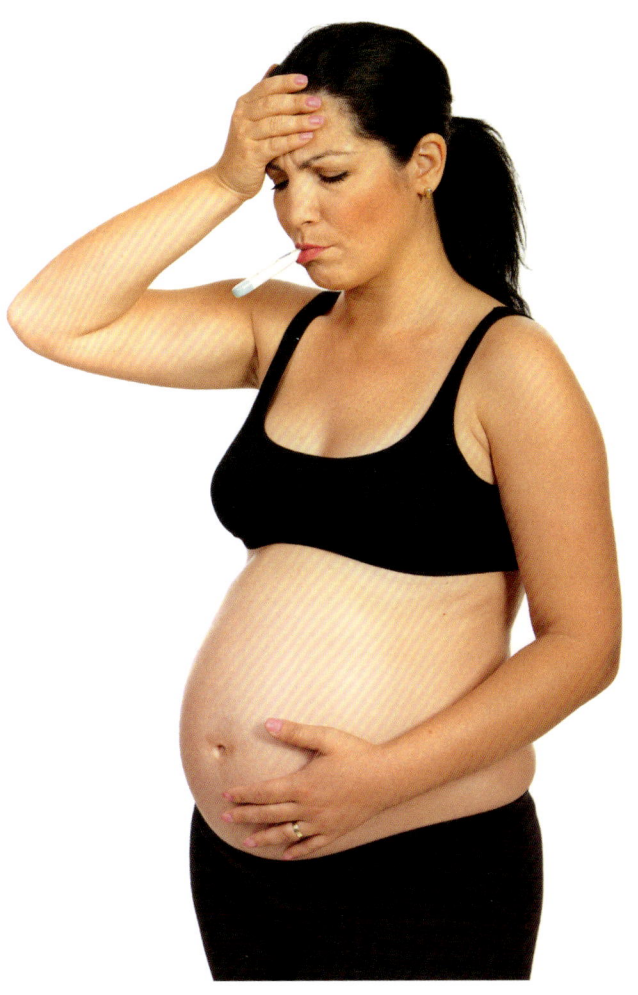

THE CHILD OR INFANT

- Beware of the septic child, infant or neonate. This group of patients are vulnerable, and often present with atypical or vague signs and symptoms. Have a high index of suspicion in these patients, and a low threshold for admission.

- Children can often compensate well during a disease process like sepsis. This means subtle changes can be missed until they suddenly decompensate and become extremely unwell.

- In young children and infants, language and understanding can be a communication barrier, you may need to take a collateral history from a parent or relative and use other means to communicate. Listen to Mum and Dad!!

- Respiratory infection and primary bacteraemia are the most common infections in children. Underlying disease and low-birth-weight in neonates, are associated with increased mortality.

- Neonates and infants have an immature immune system; this makes them at increased risk of infection. Whilst the management of the septic neonate or infant is beyond the scope of this book, special consideration is needed for management of intravenous access, fluids and antibiotics in these patients.

SUMMARY

- The treatment principles for patients with severe sepsis are identical regardless of the cause. Initial assessment and resuscitation should follow the ABCDE format with the application of the Severe Sepsis Screening Tool. Patients should benefit from the Sepsis Six, followed by the application of Early Goal-Directed Therapy where appropriate. Liaison with Critical Care should be timely, particularly in the presence of septic shock or multi-organ failure.

- Patients with pneumonia represent the largest group of patients with severe sepsis. Common causes of sepsis aside from pneumonia include gastrointestinal pathology, urinary tract, biliary tract and skin infections.

- Remember to keep an open mind when assessing a patient presenting with sepsis.

- Some suggestions for antibiotic therapy are presented above; these are intended as guidance only. The importance of consultation with microbiologists locally who will be aware of pathogens and resistance patterns in your own institutions cannot be over emphasised. Most organisations now have their recommended first-line empiric treatments for common infections on their intranet sites.

SEPSIS. SPOT IT. TREAT IT. BEAT IT.

FURTHER READING

Daniels R. Surviving sepsis. JICS 2012; 13: 10-11.

Watson RS, Carcillo JA, Linde-Zwirble WT, Clermont G, Am J Resp Crit Care Med 2003; 167 (5): 695-701

Lidicker J and Angus DC. The Epidemiology of Severe Sepsis in Children in the United States. AJRCCM 2003; 167: 695-701.

OUTLINE

During this chapter we will discuss the indications for escalating the seniority of staff or level of care for patients with sepsis/ severe sepsis, including when Critical Care involvement is required. Sepsis is a complicated condition and often requires input from several specialities such as microbiology, radiology, surgical and medical specialities. The indication for involving each of these will be reviewed. When the need for a referral has been identified the delivery and timing of this referral are crucial factors in preventing an irreversible decline in the patient's condition.

ESCALATING CARE

The Sepsis Six is a tool designed to ensure all patients diagnosed with sepsis receive early intervention to prevent organ dysfunction. It is aimed at relatively junior staff without specialist skills, and everyone in healthcare can contribute to its delivery. Despite successfully delivering these interventions, patients with sepsis remain complex and always have the capacity to deteriorate. For this reason, the most senior care provider responsible for the patient at that time should be informed about all patients with sepsis, to ensure optimal on-going care. During out of hours this is likely to be the senior registrar in the Emergency Department, or the medical or surgical registrar on the wards.

When evidence of organ hypo-perfusion; such as hypotension, raised lactate or poor urine output despite fluid resuscitation is present, patients require Early Goal Directed Therapy (EGDT). This will, for most hospitals in the UK, demand that Critical Care be involved early, since EGDT should be delivered within the first 6 hours following presentation. In some units,

Emergency or Acute Medicine teams, surgical teams and other specialist providers may have capacity to provide EGDT.

Early goal directed therapy is a bundle of care governing the initiation of invasive monitoring to guide targeted therapy aimed at restoring the circulation of patients with septic shock. It was described by Rivers et al, and demonstrated a significant survival benefit. In Rivers et al therapy was directed to reach set goals (figure 1); the first goal was to fluid resuscitate to a CVP of >8mmHg (> 12 mmHg if the patient was ventilated), once achieved the second goal was to maintain a MAP greater than 65mmHg with vasopressor support (drugs to constrict the dilated blood vessels, e.g. noradrenaline). The third goal was to maintain a central venous oxygen saturation ($ScvO_2$) >70% by optimising haemoglobin and use of inotropes (drugs to increase cardiac output, e.g. Dobutamine). The merits of these goals have been discussed extensively since, with multiple randomised controlled trials currently underway. The debate of Central Venous Pressure, $ScvO_2$ or other measures of circulatory function as the best goals in the management of severe sepsis is outside the remit of this chapter. EGDT is mentioned only to illustrate the importance of timely referral of severely septic patients to critical care. This is particularly important in patients who do not respond to fluid resuscitation, or who respond only transiently.

Severe Sepsis has a time dependant survival rate. If patients are not resuscitated early, they continue on a downward spiral of decline and mortality becomes increasingly likely (figure 2). For this reason it is important to refer all severely septic patients to Critical Care as soon as they are identified. The delivery of the Sepsis Six can then continue whilst waiting for a review by critical care. An early referral will minimise delays in relocating patients to a Critical Care unit where a physical bed space may have to be made available. If a delay is likely, outreach services can be used to ensure critical care support is given to those caring for the patient in their existing clinical area: termed 'ICU without walls'. Examples of criteria for Critical Care referral are demonstrated below (figure 3).

Whilst awaiting admission to Critical Care there is potential for conflict between the Critical Care provider and primary team as to where responsibility for the patient may lie.

This is a challenging issue as both sets of providers are likely to have other responsibilities and time constraints. Communication and the understanding that both sets of care providers have a duty of care to the patient are vital. The primary team should still ensure that the Sepsis Six has been completed fully and any ongoing fluid requirements are met. Critical Care providers should be aware of the progress of the patient and be at hand to help with difficult management decisions.

OTHER REFERRALS

As sepsis is a complicated condition it often requires a multidisciplinary approach to optimise patient management. Microbiology or Infectious Diseases teams are often available to advise on the best anti-microbial agents for septic patients. They will be able to assess information on the clinical picture, patient risk factors, current microbiology resistance profiles and the patient's culture profile to ensure adequate cover at onset of antimicrobial therapy and safe de-escalation of broad spectrum cover. When informed of patients with severe sepsis, Microbiologists will ensure that cultures are closely monitored and that the treatment adequately covers all pathogens isolated.

Medical specialities can aid in optimising the management of sepsis. Rheumatology, oncology and haematology teams are used to managing immunosuppressed patients and can liaise with microbiology to ensure all atypical infections and any non-infective causes of SIRS which may mimic sepsis are investigated for. Medical teams may also advise adding cover to protect from difficult-to -diagnose infections if they feel their patients are at risk e.g. fungaemias and TB meningitis.

One of the key factors in improving survival from sepsis is source control. This often requires a referral to an appropriate surgical speciality- e.g. a complicated dental abscess with drooling and trismus will require a referral to ENT to prevent progression to Ludwig's Angina – a potentially fatal cellulitis of the mouth floor. Often, interventional radiologists will be able to secure percutaneous drainage of abscesses, and remember that you might have a role to play in source control: removal of an infected indwelling device, such as a peripheral venous cannula, can play a crucial role in ensuring the best outcome for a patient. Source control should be achieved as soon as possible, and always within the first 12 hours following presentation.

Imaging is a key component in the diagnoses and management of severe sepsis, and even when the radiologist cannot drain a source their expertise can prove invaluable in planning surgical control. All modalities can be utilised to help diagnose the source of sepsis. Referral to a radiologist is often the least well communicated referral in a hospital system. Providing appropriate information to the radiologist and discussing complicated cases directly with them will help them provide the best modality and target their report to ensure the question being asked by the referral team is answered to their best ability.

THE ART OF REFERRING

Whether referring a patient to Critical Care or requesting additional support from senior team members or supporting specialities, the skill of communicating is very important to ensure the important information is understood and a clear expectation communicated. The failure of effective referral skills can delay time dependent interventions including EGDT.

Situation, Background, Assessment, Recommendation (SBAR) is a well-recognised mechanism to facilitate effective communication between all parts of a multidisciplinary team. SBAR is discussed in the human factors chapter but is highlighted again in case scenario 1.

Despite the use of SBAR, there will be occasions where the expectations of the referring person are not met. Sometimes, junior members of a team or other members of a multidisciplinary team recognise an impending catastrophe before the most senior. Many factors can prevent effective communication during these circumstances such as differences in experience, job position, personal power, personal agendas and fear of 'loss of face'. Graded assertiveness is a skill that provides a structured escalation of momentum to empower team members to move forward despite feeling uncomfortable doing so. An example of the use of graded assertiveness is discussed in case scenario 2. These factors are discussed in more detail in the chapter on Human Factors.

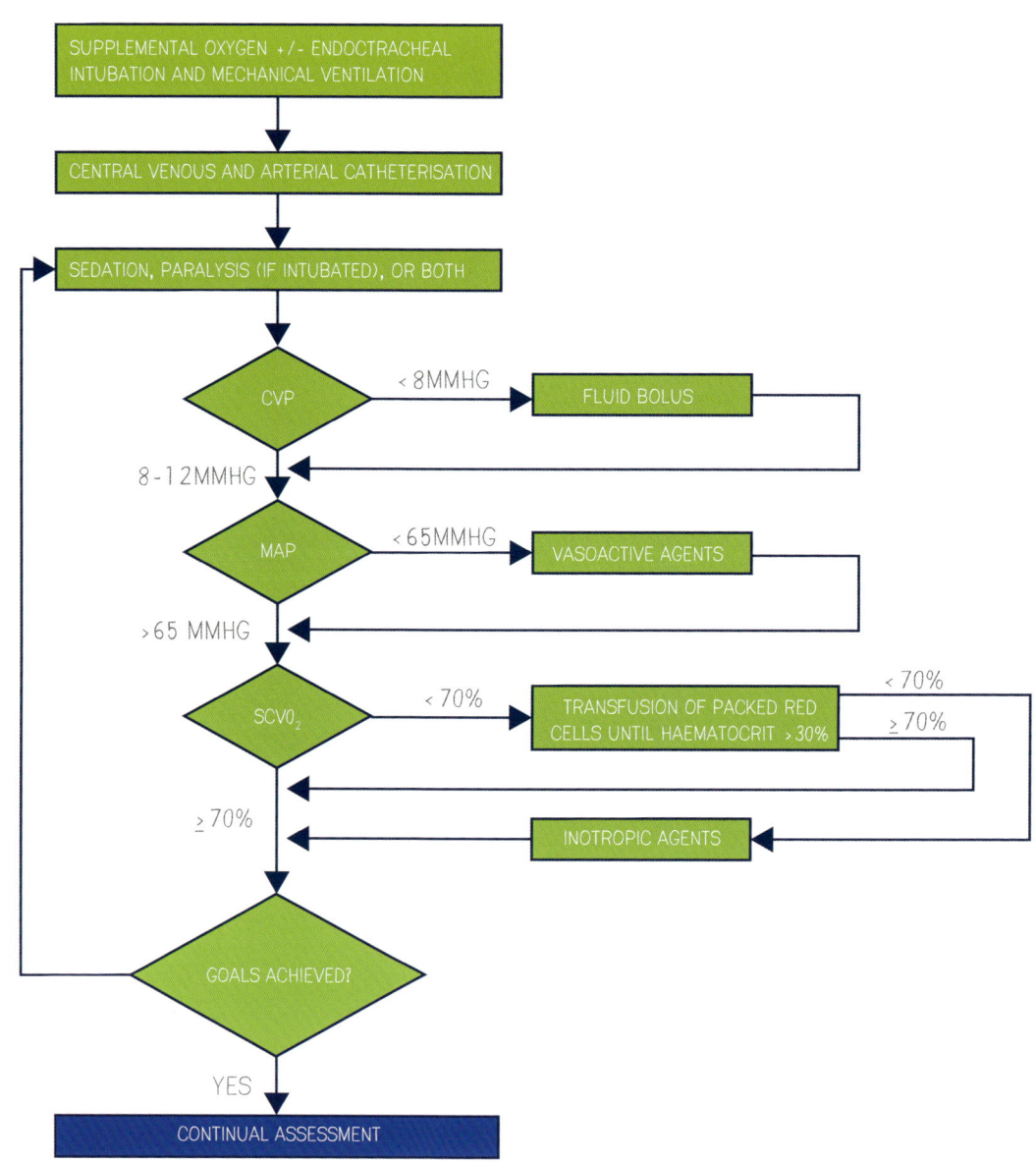

FIGURE 1: ADAPTED FROM RIVERS E, ET AL: 'PROTOCOL FOR
EARLY GOAL-DIRECTED THERAPY'. N ENGL J MED 2001.

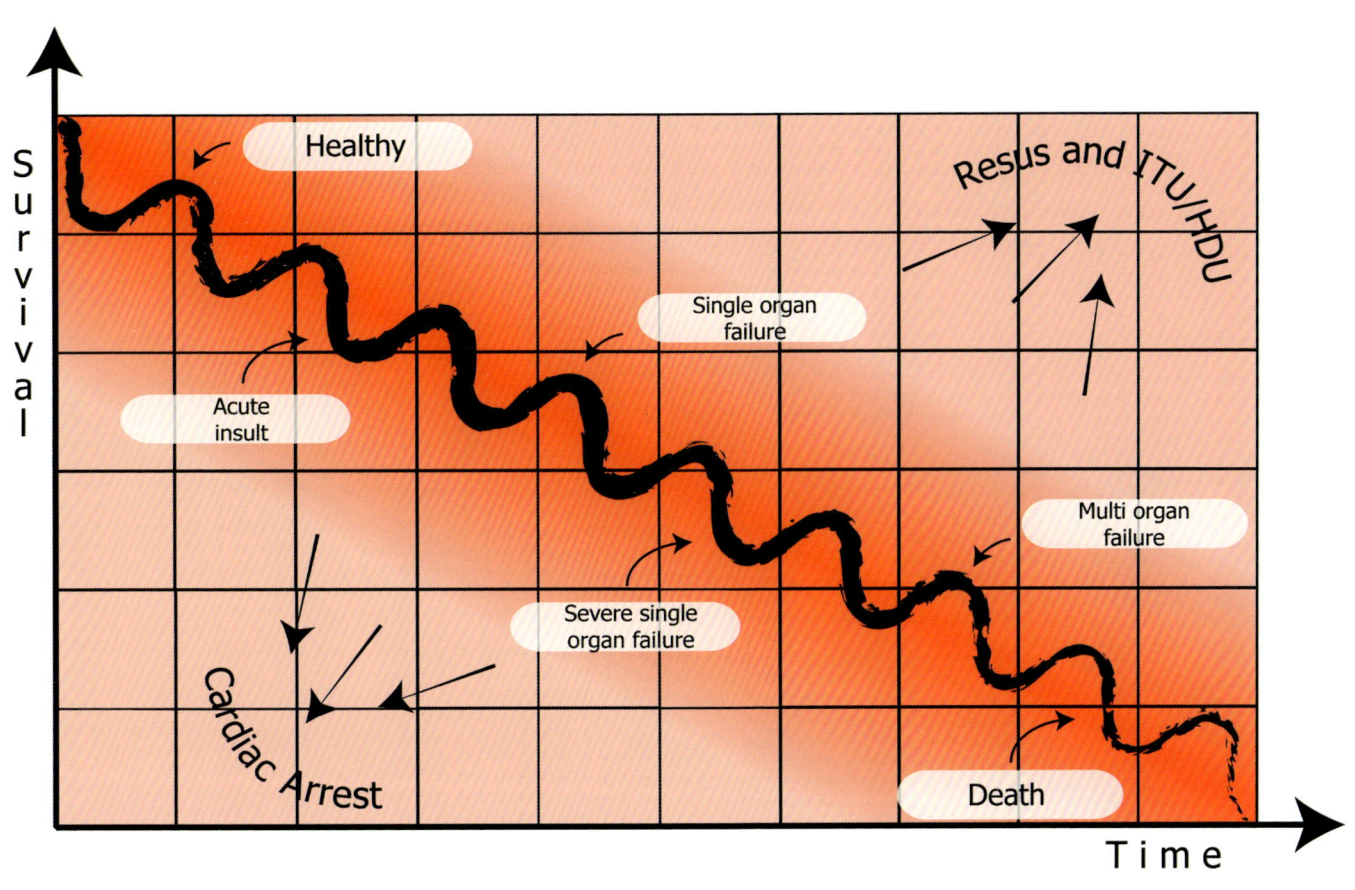

FIGURE 2: THE DOWNWARD SPIRAL OF THE SEPTIC PATIENT.

After an initial fluid bolus:

1. Is the patient hypotensive?

2. Is the patient only transiently responsive?

3. Has the patient required vasopressor support?

4. Is the serum lactate >4mmol with any of the following signs of additional organ hypo-perfusion:

    a.   Respiratory: SaO_2 <90%

    b.   Renal: urine output <0.5mls/kg/ hr for 2 hours, creatinine >177µmol/L

If yes to any of '1-4' refer to Critical Care and continue resuscitation.
If no, complete Sepsis Six and continue current management. If signs of additional organ hypo-perfusion develop, lactate fails to improve and/or the patient becomes hypotensive after 30mls/kg fluid bolus refer to Critical Care.

FIGURE 3: CRITERIA FOR REFERRING SEVERELY SEPTIC PATIENTS TO CRITICAL CARE

CASE SCENARIO 1: AN EXAMPLE OF REFERRING TO A SENIOR COLLEAGUE USING SBAR

S SITUATION: IDENTIFY YOURSELF, THE PATIENT, LOCATION AND VOICE YOUR CONCERN.

"This is Millie, the nurse on ward 3B (haematology). The reason I'm calling is that Mrs Jones in room 6 has become suddenly hypotensive, her heart rate is 110 and her blood pressure is 85/50. We have placed her on 10 litres of oxygen and started a litre of 0.9% Saline stat. She is for full and active therapy."

B BACKGROUND: GIVE PATIENT'S REASON FOR ADMISSION, PAST MEDICAL HISTORY, AND HISTORY SINCE ADMISSION.

"Mrs Jones is a 52-year-old woman admitted today with Neutropenic sepsis. She was initially febrile and hypotensive in the emergency department but responded well to antibiotics and fluid. She was assessed by ICU who felt that although she would be a candidate for ICU there was no indication at that time". She is a newly diagnosed AML patient thought to have a good prognosis. She is two weeks post her first round of chemotherapy. She has no other medical problems.

A ASSESSMENT: VITAL SIGNS, CLINICAL ASSESSMENT, CONCERNS.

"Her current vital signs are. RR 24, clear chest, saturations 99% on 6L of oxygen, HR 110 – sinus rhythm, BP85/50. She is very warm peripherally. Her GCS is E3, V5, M6. Her abdomen is soft with some tenderness over the kidneys on the left. She has passed a total of 50mls of urine in the last 3 hours. I feel that she has now progressed to severe sepsis and her condition is declining".

R RECOMMENDATION: EXPLAIN WHAT YOU NEED/WHAT YOU WOULD LIKE TO HAPPEN. MAKE SUGGESTIONS AND BE SPECIFIC ABOUT TIME FRAME.

"As the doctor covering the wards this evening, Please could you review Mrs Jones promptly and consider discussing her with your senior colleague about whether she needs to referred back to ICU".

CASE SCENARIO 2: GRADED ASSERTIVENESS TO EMPOWER MILLIE, THE WARD NURSE TO ESCALATE THE CARE OF A PATIENT

Following Millie's clear referral James, the FY1 covering the ward, arrives just as the litre of 0.9% Saline finishes. His assessment of Mrs Jones is as described by Millie earlier. James thinks that Mrs Jones requires more filling and is safe to continue with ward based care. He does not feel the need to discuss Mrs Jones with the medical registrar as she is very busy reviewing admissions to the medical assessment unit.

Millie is aware that Mrs Jones hasn't responded to the fluid challenge and continues to look more unwell. Millie undertakes the following steps of graded assertiveness:

1. **Probe:** "Did you know that Mrs. Jones has already had 4 litres of fluid in the last 5 hours?"

2. **Alert:** "I think Mrs. Jones is not fluid responsive and needs ICU care to treat her more aggressively".

3. **Challenge:** Challenge: "Mrs. Jones has septic shock and is not safe to stay on the ward".

4. **Emergency:** "Step away from the patient. I will page the medical registrar and outreach team."

HUMAN FACTORS

WHAT ARE HUMAN FACTORS AND WHY ARE THEY IMPORTANT?

In recent years, we have come to recognise that human factors play a vital role in the safe delivery of healthcare. Human factors, particularly those related to performance such as fatigue and external emotional influences, play an important role in the safe practice of technical skills. In addition to technical skills and knowledge, we need to ensure personal and team effectiveness to achieve safe practices. The other prerequisite skills for safe clinical practice are the so-called 'non-technical skills', and include behaviour, teamwork, leadership, communication and situational awareness. The lack of human factors training in the National Health Service (NHS) was highlighted after the tragic death of a patient called Elaine Bromiley during routine surgery. Her death was largely attributed to human factors. She was the wife of Martin Bromiley, a pilot who specialised in human factors training. After his wife's death, Martin focused on raising awareness about human factors to improve safety within the NHS.

The film of this case study can be viewed at:
http://www.institute.nhs.uk/safer_care/
general/human_factors.html

Human factors encompass a range of environmental, organisational and job factors that influence how we behave in our working environment. The Swiss Cheese Model of organisational accidents, proposed by James Reason, is a widely used human factors model in health care. The sequentially stacked slices of Swiss Cheese, with random holes which may permit the transition of error, in general allow no error 'through' since holes rarely align: the system, though flawed, mitigates against harm.

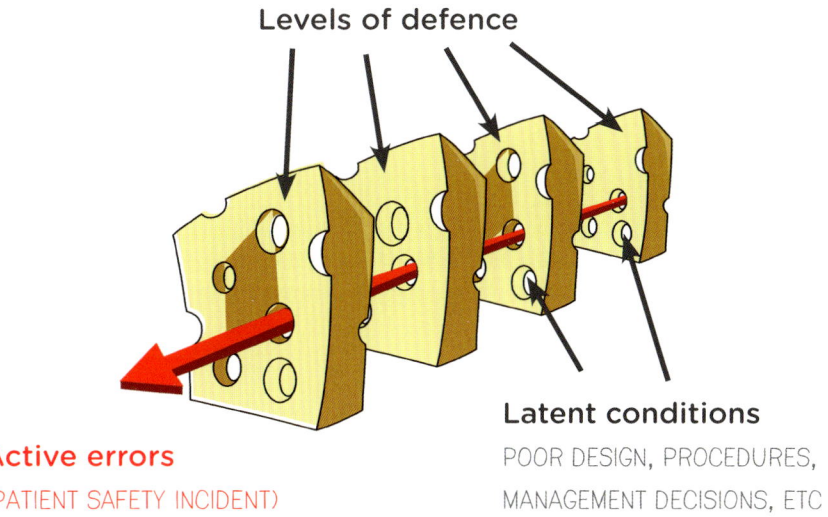

Levels of defence

Active errors
(PATIENT SAFETY INCIDENT)

Latent conditions
POOR DESIGN, PROCEDURES,
MANAGEMENT DECISIONS, ETC

THE SWISS CHEESE MODEL

In our health system we have introduced many defence levels against error, for example, checking a drug name before administration and the correct side surgery checks. However, there are holes in each level of defence which are difficult to control known as 'latent conditions': for example, poor planning, poor decision-making or poor design. A clinical incident is unlikely to occur due to one mishap-normally many small errors occur at once or sequentially on a particular day. It is these multiple failings which when aligned, like the holes in our Swiss Cheese model, breech the level of defence and a patient safety incident occurs.

We do not go to work with the intention of harming patients or causing critical incidents. However staff can often be blamed for permitting latent conditions which are often beyond their control to contribute to an adverse event. For example, in the case of drug administration, if we are stressed, under time pressure or using an unfamiliar drug, these factors can increase our risk of causing an adverse event. Applying human factors training in healthcare can improve patient safety, by helping staff to understand systems design and factors which affect their individual performance, in order to prevent these adverse incidents occurring. Thus, awareness of human factors can help identify what went wrong and what could go wrong. At the level of the organization, they can help us to gain better understanding as to why staff may make errors, and design healthcare systems and equipment to reduce the risk of errors occurring. Achieving organizational and individual awareness of human factors paves the way for the implementation of a safe, aware system and a change in organizational culture.

Human factors training can also improve teamwork and communication amongst health care workers. Working within a team and using simulation training is becoming a commonplace method of practising and testing non-technical skills amongst healthcare staff.

When managing sick patients with sepsis, many human factors contribute to the safe delivery of optimal patient care. Severe sepsis is a complex condition, often compounded by time pressures, stress and a rapidly changing environment. This is why a structured approach is needed in patient management. Multiple teams and individuals will be involved in these patients' care. Good teamwork and communication are essential to ensure the delivery of effective patient care in a timely manner.

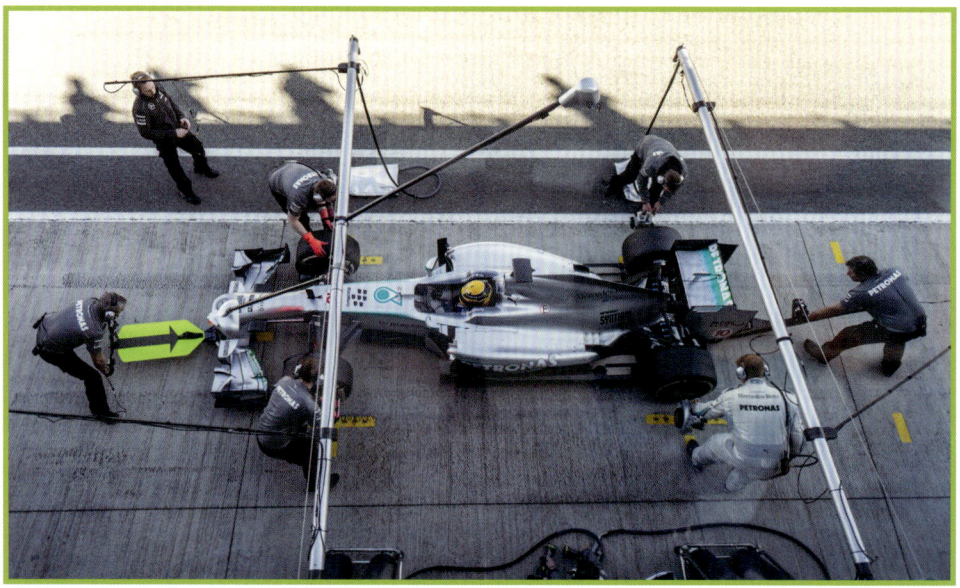

Think of a situation where you have been part of a team, managing a patient and things have gone well. Now think of a situation when things did not go so well. What factors affected the outcome in each situation? What could you have done differently to improve things?

MAKING YOUR WORKPLACE A SAFER ENVIRONMENT

We all make mistakes; as humans we cannot get things right 100 per cent of the time. When dealing with patients, as in other environments where safety is a priority, human error can both contribute to the presence of latent conditions and permit existing latent conditions to increase the risk of an adverse event occurring. There are a number of important elements involved in human factors which we can address to improve patient safety. These include: cognition, distraction, physical demands, the environment, product design, teamwork and process design.

The National Patient Safety Agency (NPSA) has produced a series of booklets called 'Design for Patient Safety' which discuss these elements in more detail. These can be found on their website.

http://www.npsa.nhs.uk/nrls/medication-zone/
design-for-patient-safety-medication-topics/.

THE CASE STUDIES BELOW DEMONSTRATE THE IMPACT OF HUMAN FACTORS ON PATIENT CARE:

CASE STUDY:

During a busy afternoon in the emergency department (ED), a 20 year old female presented at around 13.00 with a history of general malaise, left sided loin pain, urinary frequency and dysuria for the past 5 days. She was tachycardic and tachypnoeic with a temperature of 38.5°C, her blood pressure was within normal limits. Urine dipstick was positive for blood, protein and nitrites, and she was treated for sepsis secondary to pyelonephritis. Cultures were sent for urine and blood. The ED doctor prescribed a stat dose of intravenous antibiotics and one litre of intravenous crystalloid and placed the patient's drug chart in the notes slot. Meanwhile the nurse looking after the patient went on her break, which was overdue as she had already missed lunch. She asked a junior nurse to oversee her area. The junior struggled with the extra workload and did not think to check the patient's drug chart. The doctor referred the patient to the medical team, and she was promptly transferred to the medical assessment unit for further treatment without receiving fluids or antibiotics. Antibiotics were ultimately administered for the first time at 18:30, during a routine drug round.

This case highlights how an adverse event can be caused by a catalogue of smaller errors, which are often human factor-related. Think of the Swiss Cheese model.

The doctor prescribed the antibiotics and fluids correctly, however failed to communicate this to the nurse and did not delegate the task of giving the antibiotics appropriately. As there was poor communication between nurse and doctor, she may not have realised the antibiotics were prescribed or urgent. Distracted by tiredness and hunger, she goes on a break before checking this. The junior nurse may have found it difficult to voice her opinion when asked to take on extra work that she could not manage adequately, and there

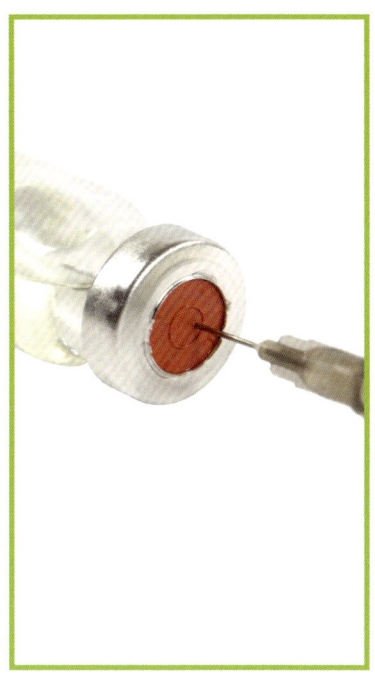

was poor handover by the nurse going on her break. There is poor teamwork and communication within this team and numerous small errors result in a critical event, whereby the patient does not receive the appropriate treatment in a timely manner: which in this case could have meant an avoidable deterioration in the patient's condition to severe sepsis.

1. COGNITION

Cognition can be affected by life's stresses, fatigue, hunger, recent alcohol or drug intake (including prescribed medication) or poor concentration. Be self-aware about these issues and take time out or ask a colleague to help you with a complex task if needed.

2. DISTRACTION

Working in a busy and dynamic healthcare setting means we have to deal with constant distractions. Distractions occur both contemporaneously (bleeps going off, a colleague asking a question) and temporally separated (a deadline for a report, problems and worries at home). The Releasing Time to Care Programme found a nurse doing a drug ward round was distracted 30 times during the round. Try to carry out difficult or complex tasks in a quiet environment, allow extra time for this and ask your colleagues not to interrupt you for a few minutes. Distractions can also be caused by busy systems; we are surrounded in patient care by care pathways and performance targets. Individuals championing these issues tend to think of their issue in isolation and design a new system around it. The result is that each new pathway or checklist tends to add to workload rather than streamline it, and has to compete with existing materials for attention. A healthy system will try to design processes to fit together.

---

3. ENVIRONMENT

Take note of your environment. Work with good lighting, keep your area tidy and organized and avoid clutter. For complex procedures, consider the use of an equipment and preparedness check list to make sure you're not missing anything. Comprehensive 'packs' containing all the equipment needed for a procedure are also useful.

CASE STUDY:

It was late at night when a 45 year old man presented to ED with a fever and productive cough. A chest X-ray (CXR) was performed which showed evidence of left lower lobe consolidation. He was diagnosed with community acquired pneumonia. He was given oxygen and cultures of blood and sputum were sent. The junior doctor had had a particularly stressful shift that night and had only recently started working in the department. She wrote the patient up for a fluid bolus and intravenous benzylpenicillin, she then remembered the patient was allergic to penicillin and quickly changed it to Tazocin®. She handed this over to the nurse to give urgently. She asked her colleague to refer the patient to the medical team and chase the blood results sent earlier, as she was meant to finish her shift over an hour ago and felt exhausted.

The ED nurse was an experienced nurse. When he went to give the antibiotics he noticed the patient's allergy status on his wristband. He had not given Tazocin® to a patient with a penicillin allergy before but he assumed the doctor must have checked this in the British National Formulary before prescribing it. As he was about to give the antibiotic the patient reminded him about his anaphylactic reaction when given penicillin, the nurse acknowledged this before giving the antibiotic.

After a matter of minutes the patient felt unwell, and developed angioedema and shortness of breath. He became hypotensive and unresponsive. He was resuscitated in ED and transferred to Critical Care for management of his anaphylaxis.

This critical event resulted due to a number of latent conditions occurring on the same day at the same time, and again there are many human factors involved here. The junior doctor is suffering from stress, both mental and physical. Tiredness could have impaired her judgement when prescribing the correct antibiotic (Tazocin® is a trade name for piperacillin with tazobactam. Piperacillin is a penicillin.). She may also have been affected by environmental factors, being new to the job. Poor communication means she does not hand over her treatment plan to the next doctor, who may have picked up on her drug error. The nurse, although experienced, does not speak up when he is unsure about the antibiotic being correct. He assumes the doctor has prescribed it correctly instead of checking for himself. No health practitioner should ever administer, or be asked to administer, a drug with which they are not familiar. Not feeling able to speak up is a common cultural barrier in hierarchal environments. Briefing and de-briefing within teams is a good way to overcome this.

4. PHYSICAL DEMANDS/ FATIGUE

A study on tiredness found that it can impact on your cognitive function and decrease your performance by the equivalent of drinking two or three beers. The 'old' system of healthcare, where juniors would work all through the night on call before commencing routine duties the next day, contributed to harm. A late night out, or being up all night with a sick relative or young child, can have the same effect. It is not a failing to admit that you're tired and ask for colleagues' support; to fail to do so might mean that you contribute to harm.

5. DEVICE DESIGN

Healthcare devices are not designed to account for human errors, and many variations of a device may be used in the healthcare setting. Minimising the variation of health equipment and ensuring staff are trained in its use can minimise the chance of errors occurring.

Think of a bank's cash point. What happens and in what order? You insert your card, provide your PIN and request your money. What happens next? The card is returned, and the money will not be delivered until you withdraw your card.

This is human factors design in action. Most of us will be focused on collecting our cash, and if the cash were delivered first the risk would be that we might leave the card in the machine and walk away.

Similarly, at a petrol station, nozzles to administer petrol and diesel are of different diameter- the system is designed to reduce the risk of the wrong fuel being used. In healthcare, our systems are often poorly designed. Drugs with opposite effects are often provided in ampoules and vials which are similar in appearance. Syringes which are designed to administer intravenous drugs can also be connected to spinal needles, although newer systems help to design this error out. The healthcare profession needs to examine its systems design, and rectify sources of error quickly.

6. TEAMWORK

Many human factors are involved in teamwork, namely communication, leadership and cultural influences. Teamwork training has been shown to reduce errors and improve performance in the Emergency Department. Briefing and de-briefing can improve communication and develop common goals and expectations amongst team members.

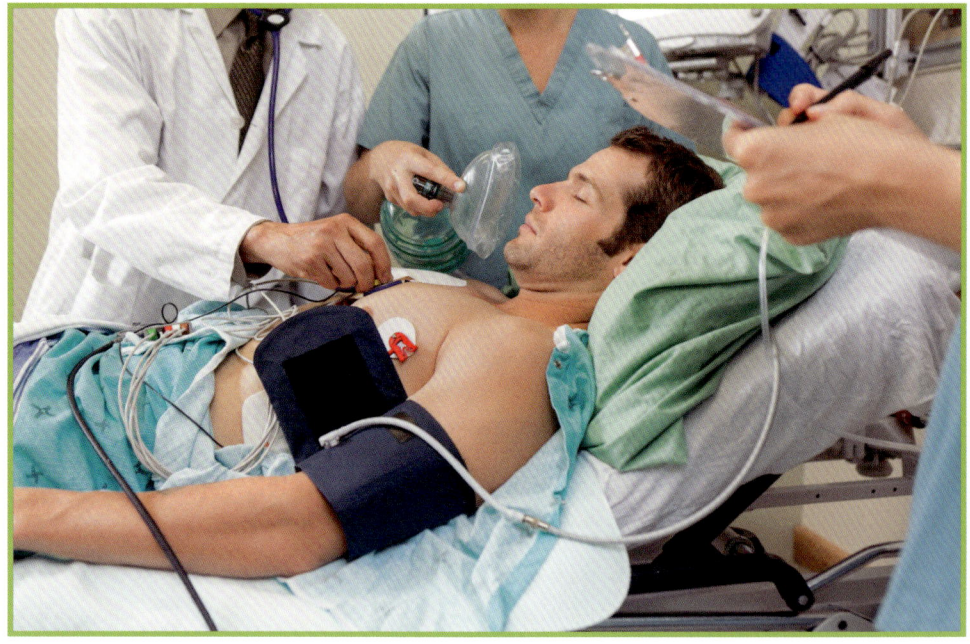

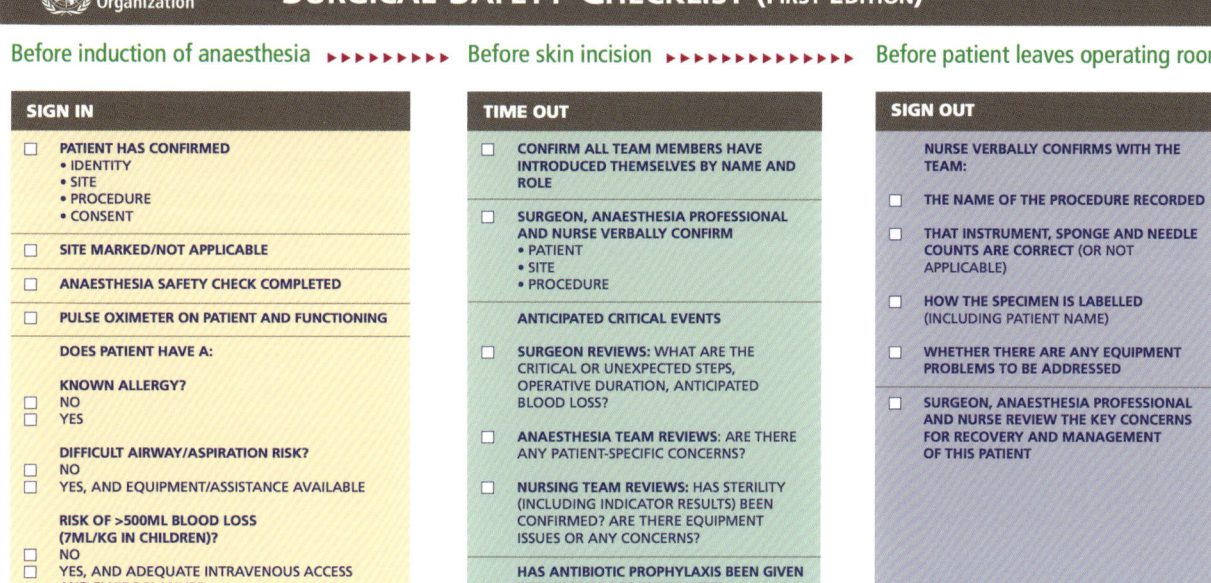

THE WHO SURGICAL SAFETY CHECKLIST
REPRODUCED WITH PERMISSION FROM THE WORLD HEALTH ORGANIZATION

Can you think of an example where this is used in clinical practice?

The World Health Organisation's (WHO) Surgical Safety Checklist is a requirement across the National Health Service (NHS), enforced by the NPSA in 2010. The checklist consists of three sections: sign in, time out, sign out, and has been shown to reduce rates of death and complications in both developed and developing countries. It is now combined with a brief and de-brief in most hospitals across the UK.

The NPSA have produced videos on how to, and how not to, use the WHO surgical safety checklist effectively. These can be accessed at:
http://www.nrls.npsa.nhs.uk/resources/?entryid45=59860

Can you think of a tool used to improve team communication?

SBAR: Situation, Background, Assessment and Recommendation

First used in the military, this tool is useful in giving a succinct handover and is often used when handing over the condition of an acutely unwell patient. This example demonstrates the tool being used effectively:

SITUATION: IDENTIFY YOURSELF, THE PATIENT, LOCATION AND VOICE YOUR CONCERN

'Good evening, is this the medical registrar with whom I am speaking?'

'Yes this is Tom Smith, the medical registrar, speaking,'

'Hello, I am Susi Hull, the Critical Care Outreach nurse coving the wards for tonight. I am ringing to discuss a patient with you who I'm concerned about. I have been asked to review an 80 year old gentleman called Jim Nicholls on ward 16. The sister on the ward called me as his MEWS (modified early warning score) is high, and he is becoming increasingly short of breath.'

BACKGROUND: GIVE PATIENT'S REASON FOR ADMISSION, PAST MEDICAL HISTORY, AND HISTORY SINCE ADMISSION

'He was admitted five days ago following a mechanical fall at home, for a fractured right neck of femur. He is usually independent, with a past medical history of controlled hypertension for which he takes Amlodipine 10mg once a day. He is also a heavy smoker. His surgery for the fracture was four days ago and has not been mobilising well since, due to pain from his hip. He has become gradually more short of breath over the past two days, and his condition has deteriorated tonight.'

ASSESSMENT: VITAL SIGNS, CLINICAL ASSESSMENT, CONCERNS

'On assessment he is drowsy and looks unwell from the end of the bed. His airway is patent, and he is tachypnoeic with a respiratory rate of 22 and course crackles at the right base on auscultation. His oxygen saturations are 88% on 4L oxygen via a facemask but he keeps pulling off the mask. His heart sounds are normal, his heart rate is 110 bpm, and his blood pressure is 90/56mmHg. He feels warm to touch and his temperature is 38.5°C, capillary refill is three seconds. He has received 125ml/hour of Hartmann's for the past 24 hours but none for the past two hours as his cannula has tissued. His urine output is borderline at 25-30ml/ hour, and he has received three doses of regular oral amoxicillin.

I have put him on 15L of high flow oxygen via a non-rebreathe mask, and re-sited a 16 gauge cannula. I have given a bolus of Hartmann's 250ml stat and his blood pressure has improved to 110/60mmHg. I have requested urgent bloods, and done a blood gas which shows a lactate of 3mmol/l. His pH is 7.30, pO_2 7.5 Kpa, and pCO_2 8.0 Kpa on the gas.

I think he has severe sepsis and respiratory failure secondary to hospital acquired pneumonia.'

RECOMMENDATION: EXPLAIN WHAT YOU NEED/WHAT YOU WOULD LIKE TO HAPPEN. MAKE SUGGESTIONS AND BE SPECIFIC ABOUT TIME FRAME

'Please could you come and review him urgently as I think he needs appropriate antibiotics prescribing, a senior review and critical care input.'

'Yes I'll be there as soon as I can.'

'Please can you give me a rough timeframe, Dr Smith, for when you can get here?'

'About ten minutes.'

'OK, thank you, would you like me to organise a CXR in the meantime? '

'Yes that would be helpful, thank you.'

7. PROCESS DESIGN:

The human memory can remember a finite amount of information. If a clinical process is too complex (for example with too many steps), this can increase the element of risk involved. However, make a process too simple and things can be forgotten.

Think about a process you have been involved with where a mistake was made. Now break this down into steps. If an important step was missed out and information did not get through, then add a step. If the process was too complex, a step can easily be forgotten so remove a step.

SUMMARY

Hopefully this brief overview has given you some insight into the importance of human factors on patient safety, and how this can translate to improved reliability in sepsis care. A collaborative approach and transparent reporting system is needed within healthcare systems with emphasis on human factors training at all levels.

Useful links:

- English Patient Safety First Campaign: guide on human factors www.patientsafetyfirst.nhs.uk

- The NPSA has a web-based programme called foresight training, aimed to develop non-technical skills amongst nurses and midwives: http://www.nrls.npsa.nhs.uk/resources/?EntryId45=59840

- The NHS justice group have produced a scope study to assess human factors training within the NHS: http://www.nhsjusticegroup.co.uk/pdf/human_factors_scoping_study.pdf
- The WHO has produced an online course: 'Introduction to Patient Safety' in collaboration with the surgical safety checklist. This can be accessed at: http://www.who.int/patientsafety/research/online_course/en/index.html

---

FURTHER READING

1. Bromiley M. Beyond technical skills: the next essential step to safety. Healthcare Risk Report 2009. Accessed 3/9/12 at http://mobilesim.files.wordpress.com/2011/03/bromiley-patient-safety-hc-risk-09.pdf

2. Reason, J. Human error: models and management. BMJ 2000; 320:768

3. Carthey J, Clarke J. Implementing human factors in health care 'how to' guide. Patient safety first 2010. Accessed 3/9/12 at http://www.patientsafetyfirst.nhs.uk/ashx/Asset.ashx?path=/Intervention-support/Human%20Factors%20How-to%20Guide%20v1.2.pdf

4. Haynes AB, Weiser TG, Berry WR, Lipsitz SR, Breizat AHS et al. A Surgical Safety Checklist to Reduce Morbidity and Mortality in a Global Population. N Engl J Med 2009; 360: 491-499

5. The NHS institute for innovation and improvement. Quality and service improvement tools: Situation-Background-Assessment-Recommendation 2008. Accessed 5/9/12 at http://www.institute.nhs.uk/quality_and_service_improvement_tools/quality_and_service_improvement_tools/sbar_-_situation_-_background_-_assessment_-_recommendation.html

CREDITS

Programme Director
Dr Ron Daniels, Chief Executive of the UK Sepsis Trust and Global Sepsis Alliance

Associate Editor
Dr Viral Thakerar - Clinical Teaching Fellow

Introduction
Dr James Cuell - Trainee in Anaesthetics

Identifying Sepsis
Dr Natalie Silvey - Trainee in ACCS/Anaesthetics

Common presentations of Sepsis Chapter
Dr Emma Joynes - Trainee in Anaesthetics

Sepsis Six
Dr Viral Thakerar - Clinical Teaching Fellow

Human Factors
Dr Emma Joynes - Trainee in Anaesthetics

Referrals
Dr Mark Sheils - Trainee in Anaesthetics

Nurse Advisor
Fiona Lawrence, Principal Educator

Illustrators
Dr. Lucia Wu - Foundation Doctor
Dr. Peter Roach
Surabhi Santosh Khanna
Dr Krupa Patel - Clinical Teaching Fellow

The Sepsis Six was created and developed by Dr Ron Daniels, Dr Tim Nutbeam, Sr Georgina McNamara, Sr Samantha Fox and Dr Katy Laver